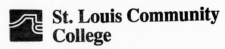

The Hearing-Impaired Child

Infancy through High School Years

The Hearing-Impaired Child

Infancy through High School Years

Antonia Brancia Maxon, Ph.D.
Department of Communication Sciences
University of Connecticut
Storrs, CT

Diane Brackett, Ph.D.
Communication Department
New York League for the Hard of Hearing
New York, NY

Andover Medical Publishers

Boston   London   Oxford   Singapore   Sydney   Toronto   Wellington

Andover Medical Publishers is an imprint of Butterworth–Heinemann.

♾ Recognizing the importance of preserving what has been written, it is the policy of Butterworth–Heinemann to have the books it publishes printed on acid-free paper, and we exert our best efforts to that end.

Library of Congress Cataloging-in-Publication Data
    Maxon, Antonia.
     The hearing-impaired child: infancy through high school years /
    Antonia Brancia Maxon, Diane Brackett.
         p. cm.
    Includes bibliographical references and index.
    ISBN 1-56372-013-2 (case bound: alk. paper)
     1. Hearing impaired children. 2. Hearing impaired children—Education.
    3. Mainstreaming in education. I. Brackett, Diane.
    II. Title.
    {DNLM: 1. Hearing Loss, Partial—in adolescence. 2. Hearing Loss, Partial—in infancy
    & childhood. 3. Mainstreaming (Education). HV 2440 M464h}
    HV2391.M28 1992
    362.4'2'083—dc20
    DNLM/DLC
    for Library of Congress   92–7050
                                   CIP

British Library Cataloguing in Publication Data
    Maxon, Antonia
    Hearing Impaired Child: Infancy Through High School Years
    I. Title II. Brackett, Diane
    371.91
    ISBN 1-56372-013-2

Butterworth–Heinemann
313 Washington Street
Newton, MA 02158–1626

10 9 8 7 6 5 4 3

Printed in the United States of America

Dedication

Sjef, Pieter and Art,
    A loaf of bread, a jug of wine, duelling laptops and thee
            T & D

Contents

Preface

Despite having a profound hearing loss that began before starting elementary school, I attended regular classes in the local public school system at a time when mainstreaming was not the norm. Although there is probably nothing in my academic record that might indicate that time spent in the regular public school system was different than a student with normal hearing, there are many incidents that occurred because of my hearing problem. Many of these incidents would have occurred even if my teachers had been fully aware of my hearing problem and knew how to deal with it. Some of the incidents, however, were problems that should have been avoided if teachers and other school officials had been better trained in how to deal with hearing problems.

At times, I could have possibly educated my teachers about assistance needed in the classroom, but even I did not have a good understanding of my hearing problem and how it affected me in school. Consequently, lack of understanding about my own hearing problem also contributed to the difficulties in school since it was not really possible to explain to the few interested teachers how I might be affected and ways of getting around the encountered difficulties.

Thomas R. Clouser

This book addresses the management of children with hearing impairment, from birth through school age (0–21 years). Management of a hearing-impaired child of any age is based on comprehensive assessment and acceptance of amplification need. Although appropriate evaluations are basic to any effective management program, they are not, by themselves, a solution to an individual's problems.

Too often assessment is strongly emphasized while management is not given the degree of attention it requires. Interpreting assessment results and developing an appropriate management plan can be difficult since speech, language, and hearing professionals have little support material to which they can refer.

Much of the research relates to information about children who are labeled "deaf" in the sense of not able to use residual hearing. Such information has minimal application to children who can and do make some use of residual hearing. Without supporting data and an understanding of the heterogeneity of the majority of children with hearing loss, professionals will continue to rely on materials that are not and cannot be adapted to a specific child. Further, these predesigned programs do not take into consideration the potential for developing an auditorally based spoken language system. This book is addressed to the many hearing health care providers and educators who, with minimal support, effectively meet the needs of their hearing-impaired students.

Throughout this book, the child with hearing loss will be referred to as the "hearing-impaired child" for reasons of style. The use of this term does not in any way reflect an attitude toward individuals with hearing loss as anything less than people first.

The Hearing-Impaired Child
Infancy through High School Years

1

Hearing Impairment

INTRODUCTION

Assessment and management of children with hearing loss is provided for under the mandates of P.L. 94-142, the Equal Education for the Handicapped Act (3–21), and P.L. 99-457, the amendment to the Equal Education for Children with Disabilities Act (0–36 months).

P.L. 94-142 provides for a variety of services for children with hearing impairment. The sections specific to management comprise "least restrictive environment" (LRE) and certain aspects of the Individualized Education Plan (IEP). Complete discussions of IEP development for children with hearing impairment can be found in Brackett (1990), and Ross, Brackett and Maxon (1991).

P.L. 94-142 has often been considered the "mainstreaming" law. As a consequence of its implementation, many children attending schools for the deaf were tra nsferred to their local public schools. The success of these moves varied with the skills of the child and the ability of the local education agency (LEA) to provide the necessary services. It is important that the relationship between "least restrictive environment" (LRE) and "most appropriate educational setting" be considered when placement and service decisions are being made. LRE is the placement that allows the child's specific needs to be met while providing maximum exposure to nonhandicapped classmates. The planning and placement team must be armed with this knowledge, a complete evaluation of the child, and a thorough awareness of the support services available within a variety of educational settings (both regular and special education). Only with a careful interpretation of LRE can decisions be made about the appropriateness of placing a particular child either in his/her "home school," within the LEA or elsewhere.

The placement options available for preschool and school-age children with hearing loss can be found in Table 1.1. These alternatives are not to be considered hierarchical with the final goal of educational management being full mainstreaming.

It is important for the child, parents, and school personnel to be aware that placement may vary from year to year, depending on the child's needs. Viewing placement changes as lateral movement allows for shifts to be made in any direction. Transitions from one educational grouping to another, e.g., preschool

Table 1.1   Educational placement alternatives for preschool and school-age children with hearing loss (Adapted from Ross, Brackett and Maxon 1991).

Mainstreaming Type	Setting	Academics	Services*
Full	Home school Central school Regular preschool	All in regular education class from regular education teacher	Auditory, Language, FM, Speech, Tutoring, Amplification monitoring
Partial	Home school Centralized school Program for hearing impaired	Some in regular education class, some in resource room/class for hearing impaired/ one-to-one	Same as above
Social	Home school Centralized school Program for hearing impaired** School for the deaf** Regular play group	All in special education class/ resource room/ class for hearing impaired by special education teacher	Same as above

*The services that are necessary depend on the individual child. Children should be candidates for FM systems and language management services.

**Requires flexibility and the ability to handle the logistical problems of transportation.

to elementary or middle school to high school, are critical times when placement decisions should be analyzed carefully relative to the student's academic, communicative, and social profile.

P.L. 99-457 mandates identification, assessment, and management services for children from birth to age three. The components of this amendment that impact on the hearing-impaired child include the development of individualized programming for the child and family through the Individualized Family Service Plan (IFSP), which is implemented by an interdisciplinary team. Acknowledging the role of the family in the management of an infant/toddler, the IFSP includes goals and objectives for the family unit. The team approach addresses the need for a broader base of knowledge when working with a very young child. The team must include a "qualified provider," the professional who best serves as the child's case manager. The professional working with the infant/toddler with hearing loss must have knowledge and skills in a wide variety of areas. Further description of the case manager is provided in Chapter 10.

No appropriate management plan, either IEP or IFSP, can be developed without very specific knowledge of a child's strengths and weaknesses. Therefore, the professionals involved must have the skills to conduct the comprehensive assessments, which cover all developmental areas for the infant or toddler who has a hearing loss.

Information on assessment of children with hearing loss can be found in Ross, Brackett and Maxon (1991); Boothroyd (1988); Ling (1976); Kretschmer & Kretschmer (1978); Moeller (1988); and Thompson et al. (1987).

It has been proposed that children with hearing loss should be viewed as a heterogeneous group with wide variance in all areas of performance—that predictions about skills cannot be made merely by knowing the type and degree of hearing loss (Ross, Brackett and Maxon, 1991). Although a programmed approach based on degree of disability may be easier, it is less effective because it is not geared to the student's particular needs.

Professionals often make generalizations based on factors other than degree of hearing loss. (Table 1.2). Although such generalizations provide a quick way to describe a group of children, they do little to further effective management strategies. The following material may help dispel the notion that categorizations are beneficial to the child and/or professional.

Hearing Loss

By definition, children with hearing impairment have hearing levels greater than 25dB HL in at least one ear. Hearing impairment, as defined by degree of hearing loss, is a continuum that spans better ear pure tone average (PTA) from 0dB HL (children with unilateral hearing loss) to greater than 110dB HL (children with minimal audiometrically measurable hearing). It is erroneous to assume that children at ei-

Table 1.2   The bases on which children's hearing loss are often grouped.

Hearing Status:	These children have hearing levels that deviate from clinically described normal limits.
Language:	The hearing loss results in language skills that are not age appropriate.
Speech Production:	An impaired auditory system decreases the ability to self-monitor production of speech.
Speech Perception:	An impaired auditory system interferes with ability to use acoustic cues to perceive speech.
Social:	Reduced communication ability interferes with development of age-appropriate social skills.
Academic Performance:	Hearing loss and language delays result in reduced academic skills.

ther end of the continuum or at any point along it have the same problems, or the equivalent ability to use their hearing.

Use of residual hearing is probably the most overlooked, underassessed, and poorly managed aspect of hearing loss. That it cannot be readily predicted from the audiogram makes it an elusive, often confusing component. It is generally true that reduced poor high frequency sensitivity negatively impacts on an individual's ability to correctly perceive consonants by decreasing the availability of acoustic cues. However, the relationship is not linear. Other factors, such as cochlear distortion, make it impossible to develop an accurate formula for predicting speech discrimination errors from hearing loss configuration. Individuals with similarly shaped audiograms can make very different use of acoustic cues, such as formant transitions. Therefore, the professional will find it crucial to carefully assess the child's use of residual hearing before developing auditory, speech, language, and educational management plans (Ross, Brackett and Maxon, 1991).

Language

It is well documented that the presence of a hearing loss will interfere with the acquisition, development, and use of language (Ross, Brackett and Maxon, 1991; Kretschmer and Kretschmer, 1978). As with use of residual hearing, it is also not possible to predict the extent of language problems merely by studying the audiogram. Clearly, the greater the degree of hearing loss and the greater the delay in fitting amplification, the more difficult it will be for the child to readily acquire language through the auditory channel. However, the literature on the language problems associated with milder degrees of hearing loss and unilateral hearing loss demonstrate that the effect often is disproportionate to that anticipated from the actual degree of loss (Bess and Tharpe, 1986; Bess, 1985). The same is true for children who have profound degrees of hearing loss. The variance in the linguistic skills must be attributed to factors other than pure tone hearing levels. Assessment of all aspects of language is basic to providing the appropriate management.

Speech Production

Developing an auditory feedback loop for self-monitoring of speech production underlies intelligible speech. Children with congenital or early onset hearing impairment will have difficulty developing this auditory feedback mechanism, unless appropriate early amplification and training are implemented. Greater access to the speech signal results in increased opportunities to develop and use the auditory feedback loop. However, even children with minimal available hearing can learn to self-monitor their speech and develop good articulation and voice quality. It is important to realize that speech production skills are directly related to speech perception, rather than to pure tone thresholds (Ross, Brackett and Maxon, 1991).

Speech Perception

Hearing loss of any degree or configuration will interfere with the development of speech perception categories. Reduced high-frequency hearing negatively affects speech perception, making it more difficult for the child to learn to use acoustic cues of speech. A child with normal hearing is consistently exposed to an audible, clear, speech signal despite interference from noise and distance, and so effortlessly acquires auditory perceptual skills. The hearing-impaired child must cope with the distortion produced by the loss and the amplification while attempting the difficult, but not impossible, task of categorizing phonemes according to their acoustic features. Early identification and auditory management will enable the child to learn to use whatever multiple cues are available through amplification.

Social

Identifying and correcting the social ramifications of hearing loss is a worthwhile goal. The professional must have an awareness of the disruptions that can occur. The research on the social aspects of hearing loss is minimal at best and often contradictory.

Children in segregated programs for the hearing impaired are found to have poorer self-perceptions than children of the same age with normal hearing. In addition, their interactions tend to be like those of younger children with normal hearing. Research on students in mainstreamed settings shows that students with greater degrees of hearing loss appear to have higher self-esteem than more mildly impaired students. Those who more closely approximate normal function seem to be more aware of their difficulties.

Maxon et al. (1991) describe the differences between preadolescent and adolescent children when grouped according to hearing status. Language ability is as important a factor as hearing loss, making it impossible to assume that children with greater degrees of hearing loss will have more difficulty than those with milder losses. While it is important to consider the possible effects of hearing impairment on a child's social skills, the professional should take care not to contaminate the results by using assessment tools that ignore the student's language competence.

Academic

Hearing loss can impact negatively on academic performance, particularly in language-based subjects. The wide variety of skills demonstrated by children with hearing impairment is not predictable from the degree and configuration of the hearing loss (Brackett and Maxon, 1986; Maxon and Brackett, 1987).

It is important to remember that all areas of performance interact. For example, a child with age-appropriate language will find it easier to interact socially and perform academically. However, the path to academic success is not easily predicted; it must be found through a carefully determined assessment plan.

SUMMARY

Hearing-impaired children present as a group with varying strengths and weaknesses. Therefore, appropriate programming that addresses individual needs must be planned by a team of professionals and parents who have information specific to the child. Management begins in infancy and continues throughout life. Flexibility is crucial since the child's needs will change as he/she matures and faces different life experiences.

References

Bess, F.H. (1985). The minimally hearing-impaired child. *Ear and Hearing* 6, 43-47.

Bess, F.H. & Tharpe, A.M. (1986). An introduction to unilateral sensorineural hearing loss in children. *Ear and Hearing* 7:1, 3-13.

Boothroyd, A. (1988). *Hearing Impairment in Young Children*. Washington, DC: A.G. Bell Association.

Brackett, D. (1990). Developing an individualized educational program for the mainstreamed hearing-impaired student. In M. Ross (Ed.) *Hearing-Impaired Children in the Mainstream*. Parkton, MD: York Press.

Brackett, D. & Maxon, A.B. (1986). Service delivery alternatives for the mainstreamed hearing-impaired child. *Language, Speech, and Hearing Services in the Schools* 17, 115-25.

Kretschmer, R.R. & Kretschmer, L.W. (1978). *Language Development and Intervention in the Hearing Impaired*. Baltimore, MD: University Park Press.

Ling, D. (1976). *Speech and the Hearing-Impaired Child: Theory and Practice*. Washington, DC: A.G. Bell Association.

Maxon, A.B. & Brackett, D. (1987). The hearing-impaired child in regular schools. *Seminars in Speech and Language* 8:4, 393-413.

Maxon, A.B., Brackett, D. & van den Berg, S.A. (1991). Self-perception of socialization: The effects of hearing status, age, and gender. *Volta Review* 93:1, 15-17.

Moeller, M.A.P. (1988). Combining formal and informal strategies for language assessment of hearing-impaired children. *Journal of the Academy of Rehabilitative Audiology* XXI, 73-99.

Ross, M., Brackett, D. & Maxon, A.B. (1991). *Assessment and Management of Hearing-Impaired Children: Principles and Practices*. Austin, TX: Pro-Ed.

Thompson, M., Biro, P., Vethivelu, S., Pious, C. & Hatfield, N. (1987). *Language Assessment of Hearing-Impaired School Age Children*. Seattle, WA: University of Washington Press.

2

Amplification

INTRODUCTION

The most basic management component for the child with hearing loss is an appropriate amplification or sensory device to make auditory signals, especially speech, available. Hearing aids and wireless FM systems will be discussed in this chapter, while sensory devices will be covered in Chapter 3.

HEARING AIDS

Hearing aids are the most common personal amplification device. There are three basic types of hearing aids: body-worn, ear-level, and in-the-ear (ITE) (including variations of each). The selection of type of hearing aid depends on the degree of hearing loss, the age, and the physical condition of the user. The following is a brief discussion of each type.

All hearing aids have several common components, which are presented in Table 2.1. The hearing aid microphone captures the acoustic signal from the air and changes it to electrical energy. That electrical signal is modified, according to the electroacoustic characteristics of the unit, and increased in intensity by the amplifier. The modified, amplified, electrical signal is changed back to an acoustic signal by

Table 2.1   Common hearing aid components and their functions.

Component	Options	Function
Microphone	Directional, Omnidirectional	Pick up acoustic signal and change it into an electrical signal
Amplifier	Low-high gain	Increase signal intensity
Transducer	Air Conduction	Change electrical signal to acoustic signal
	Bone Conduction	Change electrical signal to vibratory signal
Battery	Various disposable, rechargeable	Provide a power supply for the hearing aid

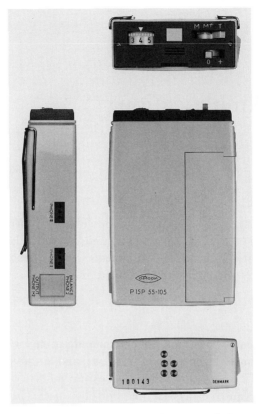

Figure 2.1   Body hearing aid. Oticon P15P body hearing aid photograph provided by Oticon Corporation, Somerset, NJ.

the transducer, and is delivered to the ear. The power source for a hearing aid is either a disposable or rechargeable battery.

Body-worn Hearing Aids

A typical body hearing aid is shown in Figure 2.1. The unit, containing the battery, amplifier, and microphone, is typically worn in a harness at chest level. The transducer, which is worn at ear level, is connected by a wire to the hearing aid. The signal from the transducer is delivered to the ear via an earmold that snaps onto the transducer. A relatively large (AA or 9-volt) battery is required to drive a body hearing aid.

Although once the hearing aid of choice for young children, and older individuals with severe and profound hearing loss, the body-worn hearing aid is no longer a common fitting. The primary disadvantages of body hearing aids are the chest-mounted (rather than ear-level) positioning of the microphone, the inadequate high frequency response, the reduced electroacoustic flexibility, and the difficulty achiev-

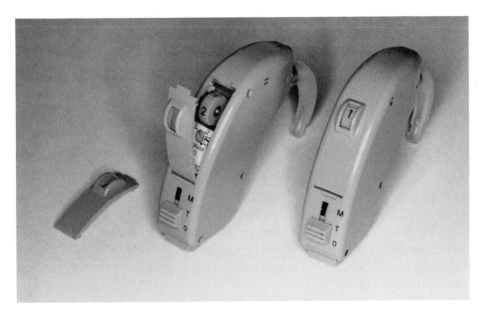

Figure 2.2   Ear-level hearing aid. Oticon E25 ear-level hearing aid photograph provided by Oticon Corporation, Somerset, NJ.

ing binaural advantages (see "Binaural Amplification" section). Although these hearing aids are durable, and have high gain and a reduced risk of acoustic feedback occurrence, it is clinically accepted that the negative factors far outweigh their advantages for most children (Maxon, 1987).

It is not just the disadvantages of body-worn hearing aids that have led to their reduced recommendation—in addition, the improvement in ear-level hearing aids has enabled that type to provide high gain (amplification). Although the possibility of feedback remains problematic with ear-level hearing aids, earmold material is now available that results in an air-tight seal between the earmold and the ear canal, thus reducing feedback (see "Earmolds" section). There may occasionally be situations in which an audiologist recommends body-worn hearing aids for infants and young children as primary amplification to increase low-frequency emphasis with the body baffle effect. (That is, the mass of the child's body reduces the amount of high-frequency sounds reaching the hearing aids because those sounds are very directional.)

Ear-level Hearing Aids

The most common fitting for children with hearing loss is the ear-level, or behind-the-ear (BTE), hearing aid (Curran, 1985). An example is shown in Figure 2.2. The microphone, amplifier, battery, and transducer are all housed in a case that fits behind the pinna (outer ear) and connects via a hook to a tube-type earmold which delivers the signal to the ear. A relatively small battery (#76, #675, #13) serves as the power supply for an ear-level hearing aid.

Ear-level hearing aids have the greatest amount of electroacoustic flexibility (see "Electroacoustic Characteristics" section). The ability to modify the way a hearing aid amplifies a signal is particularly important for infants or toddlers. A young child may be unable to provide threshold-specific information, making it necessary to change the characteristics of the hearing aid while not changing the unit itself. The way the earmold couples to the hearing aid permits earmold modifications when necessary. Since the microphones are placed at the ear, signals are received at the "normal" ear level, providing binaural advantages. Binaural stimulation is crucial for the child developing auditory perceptual skills (see "Binaural Amplification" section).

The major disadvantage of an ear-level hearing aid for young children, particularly those with greater degrees of hearing loss, is the increased likelihood of acoustic feedback. Feedback occurs when an amplified signal leaks out of the ear canal (because the earmold is not well seated) and is reintroduced to the hearing aid microphone. Closer proximity of the microphone to the transducer, and higher amplification of the signal, increase the chance of feedback. Young children are at risk because their high level of activity may loosen the earmold in the ear. Further, as they grow and their external ears change, earmolds no longer seal off the ear canal. When a child has a severe or profound hearing loss, the signal intensity being delivered by the hearing aid is so great that even a small sound leak from the earmold can produce feedback.

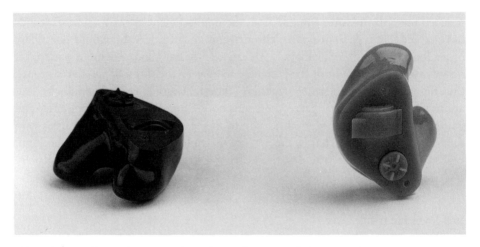

Figure 2.3   In-the-ear hearing aid. In-the-ear hearing aid photograph provided by Oticon Corporation, Somerset, NJ.

In-the-ear Hearing Aids

This hearing aid is designed to fit completely within the concha and ear canal of the individual using it (see Figure 2.3). The microphone, amplifier, transducer, and battery are all encased in an earmold that is custom made for the user—consequently, every time there is a change in earmold size the hearing aid must be recased.

The close proximity of the microphone to the transducer makes feedback a problem with in-the-ear hearing aids. In-the-ear hearing aids are typically restricted in the amount of amplification they yield, as well as in their electroacoustic flexibility.

In-the-ear hearing aids are usually recommended for individuals with milder degrees of hearing loss and for whom changes in earmolds are not common. Their usefulness for young children with hearing loss is thus limited (Curran, 1985), but children with milder degrees of hearing loss may become candidates for in-the-ear hearing aids as they get older.

A major advantage of these hearing aids is the position of the microphone in the ear, very close to the natural reception of auditory signals.

CROS/BICROS Hearing Aid

The CROS, or Contralateral Routing of Offside Signal hearing aid is designed specifically to receive the auditory signal on one side of the head and deliver it to the opposite ear. A CROS hearing aid helps overcome some of the hearing problems associated with a unilateral hearing loss (see Chapter 9). When an individual has normal hearing in one ear and a significant hearing loss in the other, it may be beneficial to deliver the signal from the poorer ear to the normal ear. However, the signal cannot be amplified because the normal ear would not tolerate it.

The CROS hearing aid looks like two individual ear-level hearing aids. However, only the unit that is worn in the poor ear has a microphone. The battery and transducer comprise the unit that is worn on the good ear. It is also possible to transmit the signal from the microphone to the transducer via a hardwire (cord) or a wireless FM arrangement. In either case, the signal is delivered to the normal ear through a specially designed earmold (see "Earmolds" section).

The use of a CROS hearing aid with children must be carefully monitored, particularly since training is required to effectively combine the routed signal and the normally arriving signal in the normal ear. The appropriateness of CROS amplification for children with unilateral hearing loss has received both positive and negative clinical reports.

A Bilateral Contralateral Routing of Offside Signals (BICROS) hearing aid is much like the CROS, except that one of the units is a complete ear-level hearing aid. BICROS amplification may be recommended when there is a significant difference in hearing between the ears. The microphone-only unit is worn on the poorer ear, while the complete hearing aid is on the better (although impaired) ear. The signal is transmitted from the microphone to the hearing aid via a hard-wired or FM arrangement, and delivered to the better ear via an appropriate earmold.

Bone Conduction Hearing Aid

All of the hearing aids discussed above couple to the ear with an earmold. For individuals whose ears cannot accommodate an earmold because of abnormalities of the ear canal or the pinna, another method of signal delivery must be used. A bone conduction hearing aid offers one such method. In a bone conduction hearing aid the transducer is a bone conduction oscillator that changes the amplified electrical signal into a vibratory one. The transducer is worn behind the ear on the mastoid process and delivers the signal via bone conduction, bypassing any structural abnormalities going directly to the cochlea. The transducer may be driven by an ear-level hearing aid, where the microphone, amplifier, and battery are all housed at ear-level, and the transducer is connected to the hearing aid by a wire and held in place with a headband. A body hearing aid also can be used to drive the oscillator.

The risk to a child of a congenital structural conductive hearing loss with obvious abnormalities of the outer ear should be known at birth. For such infants, identification and amplification should occur early since the physical malformation is visible.

Electroacoustic Characteristics

The acoustic characteristics of the signal that a hearing aid delivers are critical to the appropriateness of the fitting. The specific characteristics of each hearing aid make and model are defined by the manufacturer. The audiologist selects the characteristics on the basis of an individual's hearing loss and perceptual needs. The following is a brief discussion of some electroacoustic characteristics. A more complete description can be found in Studebaker and Hochberg, (1980).

The three basic electroacoustic characteristics of hearing aids are gain, frequency response, and output. The audiologist selects the appropriate settings through careful assessment of the individual. Most hearing aids have some electroacoustic flexibility that can be modified slightly with changing hearing needs. (See "Hearing Aid Evaluation" section for information specific to children's needs.) The process of setting the electroacoustic characteristics provides the individual with maximum access to the speech signal.

Gain

The amount of amplification (described in dB) provided by a hearing aid is referred to as gain. There are two measures of gain: reference test gain (RTG) and "full-on" gain. For both, a 60dB SPL input signal is used, and the amount of amplification is determined by averaging the intensity increase at 1000, 1600, and 2500

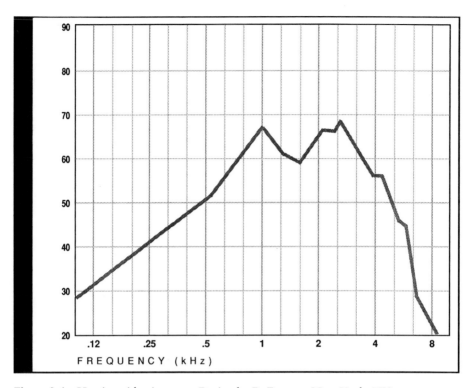

Figure 2.4 Hearing aid gain curve. Design by R. Essman, New York, NY.

Hz. A typical gain curve is displayed in Figure 2.4, where frequency (Hz) is displayed on the horizontal axis and intensity (dB gain) on the vertical axis. The two gain measures differ in volume setting; "full-on" is made with the hearing aid volume control set at maximum, whereas approximately three-quarter volume is used for RTG.

Although gain is described as a single number, it does not describe the characteristics of the whole hearing aid since only the mid-frequency range is averaged. There is no indication of amplification in the lower or higher frequencies. In order to prescribe an appropriate hearing aid, the audiologist must also know how much amplification is delivered across all frequencies. This information can be determined by using the frequency response curve.

Frequency Response Characteristics

The amount of gain provided across all frequencies can be determined by the frequency response curve of a hearing aid. A typical frequency response curve is shown in Figure 2.5, where frequency (in Hz) is given on the horizontal axis and output intensity (dB SPL) on the vertical axis. Such a curve is generated with a 60dB SPL input signal showing the output across frequencies. For most ear-level and body

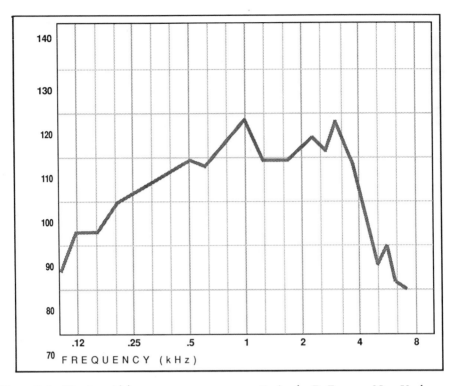

Figure 2.5   Hearing aid frequency response curve. Design by R. Essman, New York, NY.

hearing aids, gain gradually increases from the low frequencies (125 Hz) with greatest amplification in the mid frequencies, and significantly drops after 4500 Hz.

Hearing aids can be manufactured to provide a nontypical frequency response; that is, an emphasis can be given in a particular frequency region, either high or low.

Output

The greatest intensity signal that a hearing aid can provide at different frequencies is the output. The maximum output is described as SSPL-90 (saturation sound pressure level —90dB SPL input), and is measured with a 90dB SPL input signal. Output across frequencies is displayed as a curve (see Figure 2.6), where frequency (Hz) is on the horizontal axis and output intensity (dB SPL) is on the vertical axis. Although related to the gain and frequency response characteristics of a hearing aid, the SSPL-90 measure describes the maximum output that the hearing aid can produce at any given frequency when driven with a very high intensity signal. For example, a hearing aid with a gain of 45dB and SSPL-90 of 120dB at 1000 Hz will produce an amplified signal of 75dB when it receives a 35dB input.

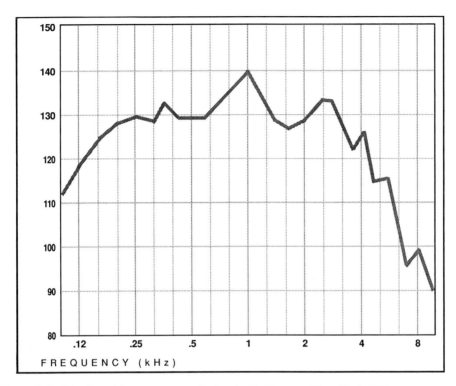

Figure 2.6   Hearing aid output curve. Design by R. Essman, New York, NY.

45 dB (Gain) + 35 dB (input signal) = 75 dB (output signal)
75 dB (output signal) ≤ 120 dB (output limit)

However, when the input is 90 dB, the hearing aid is limited by the maximum output characteristics to produce only 120 dB.

45 dB (Gain) + 90 dB (input signal) = 135 dB (potential output signal)
135 dB (potential output signal) ≥ 120 dB (output limit)

Therefore, although the hearing aid amplifies the input signal by 45 dB, the hearing aid can generate only 120 dB.

Earmolds

The earmolds that accommodate ear-level hearing aids have tubing that attaches to the hook of the hearing aid and inserts within the earmold. The canal section, which fits into the ear canal, has a sound bore that runs from the tubing insertion to an opening in the canal section.

Earmolds that accommodate snap-on transducers of body hearing aids and traditional FM systems have a metal ring that snaps onto the protrusion of the transducer button. The sound bore runs from the opening at the metal ring to the canal opening.

Earmold Acoustics

Although most hearing aids are electroacoustically flexible so that their settings can be adjusted to provide different gain, frequency response characteristics, and SSPL-90, they nonetheless have limitations. An additional means of modifying the characteristics of the signal delivered to the ear is physical modification of the earmold that couples to the hearing aid. A brief description of the most common earmold modifications follows, and is depicted in Figure 2.7

Bore

The length, diameter, and configuration of the sound bore affects the signal delivered to the ear canal. Shorter bores (0.2cm) will decrease the low-frequency components and increase the high-frequency components of the signal as compared to longer bores (greater than 1cm). Wider bores will also reduce the low frequencies, while narrower bores will enhance the highs (Lybarger, 1980). For example, a particular hearing aid will amplify less of the lower frequencies than anticipated from the

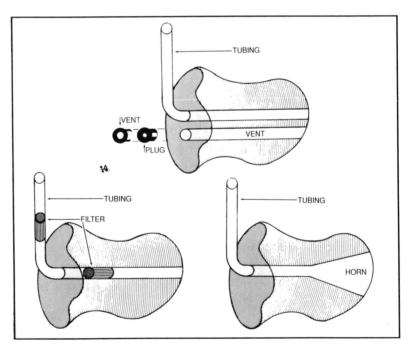

Figure 2.7   Earmold modifications. Design by R. Essman, New York, NY.

specifications when it is coupled to an earmold with a short wide bore. When the bore is flared (horn bore) at the canal opening, the modification will be an increase in high-frequency amplification.

Tubing

In nonmodified earmolds, the tubing runs uninterruptedly from the attachment at the hearing aid to the bore opening in the canal. The frequency response characteristics of a hearing aid will produce an amplified signal that will ultimately be affected by the individual's ear canal resonance. That is, the signal reaching the ear may have peaks of amplification in frequency regions different from those seen in the manufacturer's frequency response curve. These mid-frequency peaks can be reduced with a filter or damper in the tubing of the earmold, resulting in a smoother curve. The exact placement of the damper determines the specific frequency changes.

There are tubing modifications that do not affect the acoustic signal, but ensure better functioning of the hearing aid. High-gain ear-level hearing aids are more likely to have feedback problems that can be helped with extra-thick tubing. Moisture in earmold tubing can block sound or, if allowed to continue for prolonged time periods, corrode hearing aid components. Individuals who perspire in the heat or during exercise will benefit from tubing that decreases moisture buildup.

Venting

A hole can be bored in the earmold parallel to the sound bore. This vent from the ear canal to the outside allows low-frequency (longer wavelength) sounds to escape, but not high-frequency (shorter wavelength) sounds. The amount of low-frequency reduction depends on the size of the vent—the wider the vent, the greater the effect. A variable vent, one with different-sized openings, can be used to determine the best vent size for the optimum frequency response. When minimal low-frequency amplification is needed, a tube fitting can be used. Often the tubing is held in place with a skeleton mold (a ring that fits in the concha), leaving the concha and ear canal open. This fitting affords maximum reduction of low frequencies with the greatest possible "venting."

The information about earmold modification effects derives from research with adults. Extrapolation of these effects to the smaller pediatric ear is difficult. For example, the impossibility of increasing the width or length of the bore or providing a flared opening (horn bore) creates potential problems. Careful assessment of the effects of earmold modifications must be made when working with the infant, toddler, or young child with hearing loss (see "Hearing Aid Evaluation" section).

Binaural Amplification

All children with bilateral hearing losses are candidates for binaural amplification. A great deal of information is available on the pros and cons of binaural amplification (Libby, 1980), especially with the pediatric population (Maxon, 1977; Maxon, 1981).

Binaural amplification can provide binaural advantages similar to those achieved by individuals with normal hearing or relatively equal hearing bilaterally. Such advantages include the ability to localize the source of a sound, improve speech perception in a background of noise, and perceive auditory spatial relations (Libby, 1980).

Although pediatric research is sparse, it has been shown that children with hearing loss can make use of interaural cues with various types of binaural amplification (Maxon and Mazor, 1977; Maxon, Brackett, Zara, and Ross, 1988). Young children vocalize more, localize better, and have better spatial perception when using binaural amplification (Levitt and Voroba, 1980). Further, it has been demonstrated that when children have bilaterally symmetrical hearing losses and use monaural amplification, the auditory abilities of the unamplified ear deteriorate (Markides, 1977; Ross, 1977). For these reasons, it is important to provide binaural amplification to infants/toddlers as soon as they are identified so that any possible negative effects of less-than-optimal amplification can be avoided.

There are professionals who question a binaural fitting when complete audiometric information is not available. Although such concerns should be considered, they should not inhibit a binaural recommendation (Maxon, 1987).

Selection and Fitting

Personal amplification is crucial for children with hearing loss, regardless of type or degree. The audiologist must decide on the particular type, make, or model of hearing aid or sensory device, but there should be no question about the need for amplification. Any other decision would mean that the child would not have access to auditory signals, including speech. Access to the auditory signal is requisite for effective, appropriate management of the hearing-impaired child (see Chapters 4–7).

Rarely is there any question or concern about recommending hearing aids for children with moderate or severe degrees of sensorineural hearing loss. However, children with hearing levels at either end of the hearing loss continuum, i.e., mild or profound, are not always afforded the opportunity to maximize their residual hearing. Because they can "hear" without amplification, children with mild hearing loss may not receive the audiological management required for them to reach their potential. Professionals and families may assume that because their hearing levels are close to normal on the audiogram they do not need services as do children with greater degrees of hearing loss. (See Chapter 9 for a discussion of children with mild hearing loss.)

It is often assumed erroneously that the child with a profound hearing loss has too little hearing to benefit from amplification. The gains that can be made with minimal residual hearing are discussed in Chapter 4. Children who cannot

Table 2.2 Practical problems in maintaining hearing aid use and suggested remedies.

Problem	Suggested Remedy
Maintaining an ear-level hearing aid on the ear	Huggie Aids, Sports Eye Glass Holder
Batteries are removed	Battery door lock
Volume is changed	Control cover
On/Off switch is changed	Control cover
Food/liquid in top-mounted microphone on a body aid	Microphone cover
Cords pull out of jack	Replace with longer ones
Earmolds pull off hearing aid	Replace earmold, replace tubing

benefit from traditional amplification may be given access to an auditory signal through a sensory device (see Chapter 3).

Selecting and fitting optimal amplification is only accomplished following careful assessment and observation. However, even the most appropriate hearing aids will not be beneficial if there are practical problems with maintaining daily use patterns. Some of these problems (and their solutions) are presented in Table 2.2.

WIRELESS FM SYSTEMS

Although personal hearing aids can provide access to the speech signal in optimal listening conditions, there are times when interference with the signal will make listening through a hearing aid quite difficult. Certain conditions—distance from the sound source, relatively high levels of background noise, and long reverberation times—decrease an individual's ability to perceive speech through amplification (Ross and Giolas, 1971; Finitzo-Hieber and Tillman, 1978; Ross, Brackett, and Maxon, 1991). Such negative listening conditions result from a poor signal-to-noise ratio (S/N), the causes of which vary. Distance from the sound source reduces the signal intensity reaching an individual's amplification. The negative effect of background noise that is as loud as or louder than the signal will be exacerbated by amplification. Reverberation time—the amount of time a sound continues to propagate after the source has stopped—also contributes to background noise by prolonging the vowels relative to the consonants. In general, a negative signal-to-noise ratio indicates that the speech is not loud enough to be separated from the ambient noise in a room, making speech discrimination difficult. Specifically, any poor listening condition has a disproportionately negative effect on individuals using amplification.

To attain an optimal speech discrimination score, hearing-impaired children need a signal-to-noise ratio of at least +20dB; that is, the speech must be 20dB louder

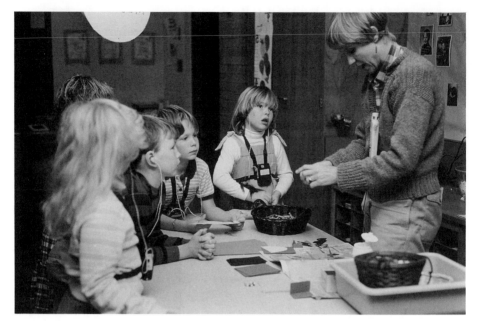

Figure 2.8   Traditional FM unit. Telex TDR-7 FM unit photograph provided by Telex Corporation, Minneapolis, MN.

than the background noise. If a speech signal is 65 dB SPL/45 dB HL (normal conversational speech level) and the background noise is 60 dB SPL/40 dB HL (average ambient noise level in a classroom), the S/N equals +5dB. Since this would not be good enough for the individual with hearing loss, the signal-to-noise ratio would have to be improved by either increasing the level of the speech signal or decreasing the ambient noise level. In the example, increasing speech would be difficult since it is at a normal conversational level.

Some negative listening conditions can be overcome by physical modification of a room (use of sound-absorbent material) to decrease noise, and/or by decreasing the distance between the child and the speech source. However, the most effective and efficient method of improving the signal-to-noise ratio is the use of a remote microphone near the sound source, as in a wireless FM auditory system. FM systems were initially designed to improve the listening environment for school-age children with hearing loss. There is recent evidence that an FM system used as primary amplification can benefit the child with severe to profound hearing loss (Madell, in press). The following is a brief discussion of FM systems and how they overcome difficult listening conditions (see Chapters 5–7 for further information on FM use.)

Traditional FM Systems

An FM system has two basic components: a microphone/transmitter and an amplifier/receiver. An example of a traditional FM system is seen in Figure 2.8. In the traditional system the transmitter is used at the sound source. It is a remote microphone that picks up a signal from the air, or via direct electrical input, and transmits it on a carrier wave (in this case a frequency-modulated [FM] signal). This radio frequency is set so that it can be received only by a unit that is specifically tuned. The system functions like a common household radio, which receives a station broadcasting a signal when it is set to the correct frequency.

The FM receiver has a dual purpose: it serves as a radio frequency receiver, and as a hearing aid with its own microphones (environmental), amplifier, and transducers. The environmental microphones pick up signals from the air so that users can hear background sound, speech of others, and their own speech. The signal delivered to the ear is a combination of the signal from the environmental microphones (background sound) and the transmitter (sound source), with the latter signal maintained at a greater intensity than that from the environmental microphones. Using the microphone/transmitter ensures a positive signal-to-noise ratio because of the relationship of the signals from the transmitter (sound source) and the environmental microphones (background noise), and because the transmitter is always close to the sound source, eliminating the distance factor.

The receiver of a traditional FM system is much like a body-worn hearing aid. It is typically worn at chest level, and the signal is delivered to snap-on transducers via wires (see Figure 2.8). It differs from a hearing aid because it has two channels (essentially two hearing aids) combined in the unit. The electroacoustic characteristics of the FM receiver must be carefully selected and set for the user. The two channels require that the settings be determined for each ear individually. Special care must be taken when the ears are asymmetrical; that is, have different hearing levels and/or configurations of loss.

The traditional FM system is commonly recommended for younger school-age and preschool-age children with hearing loss. It may also be chosen when an FM unit is used as primary amplification. Older children may find a chest-mounted FM system with wires and snap-on transducers unappealing, preferring one that is smaller and makes use of their hearing aids.

Alternative FM Couplings

As FM systems became more common in regular education classrooms in the 1980s, manufacturers developed units that could be utilized with an individual's personal amplification. Various couplings were manufactured; the two most common ones were direct audio input and the induction loop. Both devices are shown in Figure 2.9.

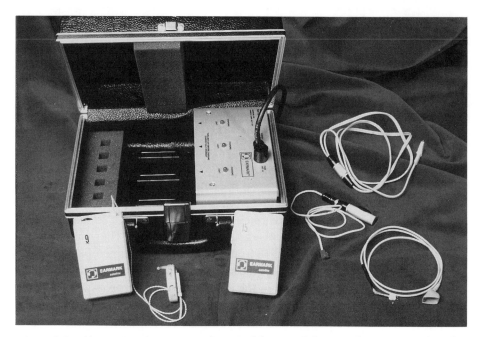

Figure 2.9   Alternative FM unit couplings. Teleloop and direct audio input coupling for Earmark FM system provided by Earmark Corporation, Hamden, CT.

Their major difference from traditional FM units is that they deliver the signal, to the ear via a personal hearing aid instead of a snap-on transducer. In this way, the electroacoustic characteristics of the hearing aid may be exploited along with the FM system. Regardless of selected coupling method, the FM unit has two components: the microphone/transmitter and the receiver.

Direct audio input coupling is a wire connection from the FM receiver to the hearing aid (see Figure 2.9). The connector is either a plug into the adapted hearing aid, or a "boot/shoe" that slips over the hearing aid to an electrical connection. Hearing aids must be specially designed to accommodate direct audio input. Therefore, the need for this type of FM coupling must be considered when a hearing aid is recommended.

Use of an induction loop coupling requires that a hearing aid have a telecoil. There is no hardwire connection, but a teleloop is worn around the neck. The loop sets up a small magnetic field from which a signal can be received by the hearing aid telecoil placed within the field. The signal is modified, amplified, and changed to an acoustic signal by the hearing aid, and then delivered to the ear via the earmold. (Detailed information on FM systems and various coupling methods may be found in Ross, Brackett, and Maxon, 1991 and Ross, in press.)

Coupling the FM system via the hearing aid was a method developed to provide a more consistent auditory signal to the child by modifying the final electroacoustic signal through the hearing aid and possibly modified earmolds. Research has demonstrated, however, that combining the two systems may produce some negative interactions.

Hearing aid telecoils typically do not have the same electroacoustic characteristics as microphones. Therefore, although the hearing aid microphone may provide appropriate amplification, the telecoil may not be adequate. Some manufacturers now provide information about the electroacoustic specifications of a hearing aid telecoil, but gain, output and frequency response should nonetheless be measured when coupled to the FM system. Further, the output and linearity of the amplification may be compromised and distortion increased when either a teleloop or direct audio input is used (Hawkins and Van Tassell, 1982; Hawkins and Schum, 1985; Thibodeau, McCarthy, and Abrahamson, 1988; LeMay, 1991).

Professionals working with children who use either direct audio input or the induction loop and telecoil must be aware of issues that may compromise FM use. For the school-age child, incorporating the hearing aid into the school-worn amplification means that a nonfunctioning hearing aid results in a nonfunctioning FM system. A backup system must be available when problems arise. For example, cords, snap-on transducers, and earmolds may be used while the hearing aid is being repaired.

The purpose of an FM system is to overcome the difficult listening conditions caused by negative signal-to-noise ratios. This function may be difficult for families, children, and school personnel to understand. A careful demonstration can convince the professionals responsible for purchasing and using the system as well as the child and family. An outline for demonstrating the benefits of an FM system for school-age children is given in Chapter 7. These methods may be used prior to the initial FM recommendation, or when the child changes educational setting or FM type. Demonstration may also be necessary when there is concern regarding either the necessity for continued FM use or the benefit received in a particular setting.

Monitoring

Monitoring amplification is a basic yet crucial aspect of managing children with hearing loss. Careful monitoring of a child's amplification performance is important in both the initial and ongoing validation of personal and school-worn amplification. An amplification monitoring checklist (see Appendix) assists families and school personnel in evaluating amplification use. Decisions about the appropriateness of the amplification in the child's various listening environments can be based on the information on the checklist.

Educational personnel and families may not be aware that even the most appropriate hearing aids and FM system cannot provide optimal listening in all situations. Regular monitoring is the only method of validating a child's performance in daily living conditions. Although the dispensing audiologist will have taken care to make the best possible electroacoustic recommendations, the restricted conditions of clinical assessment do not allow for evaluation in less-than-optimal listening conditions.

Monitoring performance must go beyond obvious auditory changes. For example, a child who previously used past tense markers (/t/ as in "walked") consistently may begin omitting them. For this child, the higher end of the amplification's frequency response curve may have changed, causing an inability to self-monitor production of the voiceless sound. A younger child may have similar problems that are manifested as an inability to repeat some of the Ling 5-sounds. The speech-language pathologist working with this child must differentiate between auditory-related and language-related problems. To do so, he/she must be well acquainted with the child's linguistic, speech production, and auditory skills. Otherwise, the clinician may assume that the child does not know the syntactic rule, when in fact he/she does know the rule, but is having an amplification problem that can be remedied.

This aspect of amplification monitoring and validation is invaluable to the audiologist. Information such as speech production and self-monitoring problems would not be available to him/her without the input of someone like the school speech-language pathologist.

Troubleshooting

Daily amplification troubleshooting should be an integral part of every child's management program. The troubleshooting schedule, the professional designated to conduct it, the method of repair, etc., should all be described in the IFSP and IEP. A summary adapted from Ross, Brackett and Maxon, (1991) is provided in the Appendix. An effective troubleshooting program includes a clear outline of the method for correcting problems. The designated professional/family member should have a supply of spare batteries, cords, and transducers to replace those that are not functioning properly, as well as tools for cleaning the earmolds, and a contact for carrying out repairs that cannot be made on site.

An effective troubleshooting program allows for checking amplification on demand as well as during the daily monitoring session. That is, a listening check should be conducted when a problem is reported, regardless of equipment status at the start of the day. Amplification must also be checked immediately prior to all assessments (e.g., communication, educational) to remove any doubt about the effect of amplification function on test performance.

Troubleshooting an FM with alternative coupling requires that the designated professional be aware of how the FM couples to the hearing aid. Further, he/she must know how to separately assess the function of the hearing aid and FM unit and the child's performance with both.

Although education of parents and school personnel is a basic component of an effective troubleshooting program, the role of the child should not be overlooked. Troubleshooting should never be the sole responsibility of the child, but he/she can be involved to some degree depending on age, degree of hearing loss, and auditory skills. For example, even children with significant hearing losses can report when the battery is dead. It is never too early to start training children to report any problems in amplification function or inappropriate use by others.

COMMUNICATION AMONG PROFESSIONALS AND WITH FAMILIES

A need for open communication between professionals and families and among professionals is always needed. Managing the child with hearing loss requires that different professionals work with the child and family. Further, the program may be carried out through different methods (e.g., child-directed, family-directed) and different settings (e.g., clinic-based, home-based). Therefore, although the content remains the same for a given child, the type and level of information exchanged will vary across interactors, method, and setting.

The scope of shared information is wide, requiring a range of interaction levels. The information must include a complete description of the child's amplification including the electroacoustic specifications and settings, types of earmolds including any modifications, performance expected from the child, and expected difficulties in various settings. Detailed information about different age groups is presented in Chapters 5–7.

SUMMARY

Regardless of communication modality, reception of speech plays an important role in managing a hearing-impaired child. Amplification provides the raw material for developing an auditory-based spoken language system. Other sensory devices should be explored when sufficient benefit is not attainable through a traditional system.

References

Curran, J.R. (1985). ITE aids for children: Survey of attitudes and practices of audiologists. *Hearing Instruments* 36:4, 20-25.

Finitzo-Hieber, T. & Tillman, T.W. (1978). Room acoustics effects on monosyllabic word discrimination for normal and hearing-impaired children. *Journal of Speech and Hearing Research* 21, 440-458.

Hawkins, D.B. & Schum, D.J. (1985). Some effects of FM system coupling on hearing aid characteristics. *Journal of Speech and Hearing Disorders* 50, 132-141.

Hawkins, D.B. & Van Tassell, D.J. (1982). Electroacoustic characteristics of personal FM systems. *Journal of Speech and Hearing Disorders* 47, 355-362.

LeMay, M.W. (1991). The effects of FM signal modification controls on the output of a personal FM system. Unpublished M.A. thesis. Storrs, CT: University of Connecticut.

Levitt, H. & Voroba, B. (1980). Binaural hearing. In E.R. Libby (Ed.) *Binaural Hearing and Amplification, Vols. I and II* (pp. 59-80). Chicago, IL: Zenetron Corporation.

Libby, E.R. (1980). *Binaural Hearing and Amplification, Vols. I and II.* Chicago, IL: Zenetron Corporation.

Lybarger, S.F. (1980). Earmold modifications. In G.A. Studebaker & I. Hochberg (Eds.) *Acoustical Factors Affecting Hearing Aid Performance* (pp. 197-217). Baltimore, MD: University Park Press.

Madell, J.R. (in press). The FM system as an initial amplification device. In M. Ross (Ed.) *FM Auditory Training Systems.* Parkton, MD: York Press.

Markides, A. (1977). *Binaural Hearing Aids.* New York, NY: Academic Press.

Maxon, A.B. (1981). Binaural amplification of young children: A clinical application of Ross' theory. *Ear and Hearing* 2:5, 215-219.

Maxon, A.B. (1987). Pediatric amplification. In F.N. Martin (Ed.) *Hearing Disorders in Children* (pp. 361-395). Austin, TX: Pro-Ed.

Maxon, A.B., Brackett, D., Zara, C. & Ross, M. (1988). Children's localization abilities: Effects of age, hearing loss, and amplification. Paper presented at the American Speech-Language-Hearing Association Convention, New Orleans, LA.

Maxon, A.B. & Mazor, M. (1977). The effects of microphone spacing on auditory localization. *Audiology* 16:5, 438-445.

Ross, M. (1977). Binaural versus monaural hearing aids. In F.H. Bess (Ed.) *Childhood Deafness: Causation, Assessment and Management* (pp. 235-249). New York, NY: Grune and Stratton.

Ross, M. (in press). *FM Auditory Training Systems.* Parkton, MD: York Press.

Ross, M., Brackett, D. & Maxon, A.B. (1991). *Assessment and Management of Mainstreamed Hearing-Impaired Children: Principles and Practices.* Austin, TX: Pro-Ed.

Ross, M. & Giolas, T.G. (1971). Effects of three classroom listening conditions on speech intelligibility. *American Annals of the Deaf* 116, 580-584.

Studebaker, G.A. & Hochberg, I. (1980). *Acoustical Factors Affecting Hearing Aid Performance.* Baltimore, MD: University Park Press.

Thibodeau, L.M., McCaffrey, H. & Abrahamson, J. (1988). Effects of coupling hearing aids to FM systems via neckloops. *Journal of the Academy of Rehabilitative Audiology* 21, 49-56.

3

Alternative Sensory Aids

INTRODUCTION

The majority of children with permanent sensorineural hearing loss will be accommodated by the traditional forms of personal and school-worn amplification described in the preceding chapter. However, there are some children for whom such devices do not provide an appropriate signal. Depending on the type and degree of loss the child demonstrates, an alternative type of sensory device may be more beneficial.

The most obvious example is the child with bilateral profound sensorineural hearing for whom hearing aids and/or FM systems cannot deliver a signal intense enough to make auditory stimuli (particularly speech) audible. For these children, access to the speech signal can be achieved through a cochlear implant or a vibrotactile device.

Children with very mild sensorineural hearing loss, or those with fluctuating conductive hearing loss, may benefit from a more positive signal-to-noise ratio than typical. For these children, a device such as a sound field FM system may be particularly useful, either with or without personal amplification.

All hearing-impaired children, regardless of degree of hearing loss or ability to use traditional amplification, may be candidates for assistive devices that present speech in an acoustic or supplemental visual form. Such devices allow the child to use a signal delivered, for example, over the telephone, the television, or in a large auditorium. Careful use of these systems in conjunction with a regular amplification or sensory device can allow the child to learn from and interact in a wide variety of listening conditions.

COCHLEAR IMPLANTS

Cochlear implant use for children began in the early 1980s, after a long history with profoundly hearing-impaired adults. The initial device was a single-channel electrode inserted 6 mm into the cochlea that stimulated a small area at its base. The children who used this single channel implant demonstrated improved detection of speech patterns, with only a very small number of them able to recognize words in

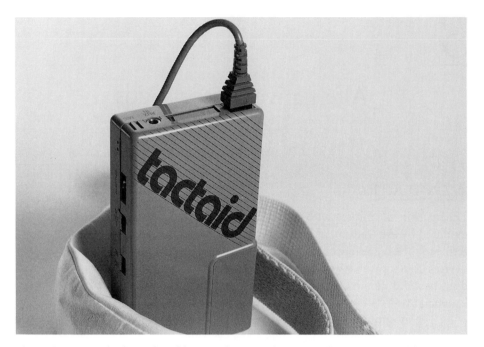

Figure 3.1   A multichannel cochlear implant. Nucleus 22 with MSP provided by Cochlear Corporation, Englewood, CO.

an open-set task. This exciting beginning provided the impetus for further developments in implantable auditory devices that continues to this day.

In 1987, the U.S. Food and Drug Administration (FDA) placed the Nucleus 22 multichannel implant on investigational status for use with profoundly deaf children ages two to seventeen years, following a successful trial period with adults. This device has few features in common with the single-channel implant of the early 1980s. The acoustic signal is initially transformed by an external microphone into electrical energy and is transmitted via a radio signal across the scalp to the subcutaneous receiver, where it is sent to the 22-electrode array. The internal components of the 22-channel device consist of a receiver that is anchored under the scalp in an indentation in the skull (mastoid process) directly behind the ear. The electrode is fed one and one-half turns into the cochlear near the CN VIII nerve endings. Electrode #1 is the furthest in distance from the round window and Electrode #22 the closest. As seen in Figure 3.1, the external components include an ear-level microphone connected via a cord to a speech processor—either the WSP (wearable speech processor) or the newer MSP (mini speech processor), which sends the signal to a transmitter attached to the scalp with a magnet. (Figure 3.1a.)

Rather than taking the speech signal as it exists, the speech processor uses a coding strategy that extracts the first and second formants of vowels, as well as the primary energy regions of the consonants (Koch et al., 1990). The frequency-specific information from the speech processor is divided among the 22 electrodes, which have been assigned specific frequency ranges: for example, on a specific child's map, #1 may be responsible for 1-200 Hz, #10 assigned 1000-2000 Hz, and #22 set for 3000-4000 Hz. The fundamental frequency of the voice is determined by the rate of stimulation. Loudness is determined by the amount of current delivered to each electrode.

The FDA approved the clinical use of the multichannel cochlear implant in June 1990 for profoundly deaf children, ages two to seventeen years who are unable to benefit from traditional amplification. Candidacy is determined by a multidisciplinary team that assesses the child's auditory, communicative, and psychosocial functioning. Factors such as motivation, demand to listen, school involvement, availability of services, and parental commitment all enter into the decision-making process. The child's communication mode is not an exclusionary factor as long as an auditory emphasis is included in the child's educational/rehabilitative program. Currently, 53.6% of the implanted children nationwide use *Total Communication*, 33.8% *Auditory-Verbal*, and 12.5% *Cued Speech*. The long-term nature of the rehabilitation and follow-up should be considered by the family, child, and implant team when deciding to proceed with an implant.

As of early 1991, over 500 children had been implanted. All of the children detected sound at normal conversational levels. Some are able to understand speech using only the sound received through the implant. Many others can identify words without lipreading when given a limited choice. Their ability to receive speech using full auditory and visual input has improved dramatically. The communication skills of all the children have also improved. Increased speech intelligibility is a realistic expectation for many children.

As of January 1991, 61% of the children who have been implanted are in self-contained classes in public schools or in schools for the deaf, reflecting the typical placement for profoundly hearing-impaired children in the United States. Although the teachers in self-contained classes are knowledgeable about the needs of hearing-impaired children, they require in-service training about the expected performance parameters of children with cochlear implants. The children in self-contained classes have a long history of nonauditory interaction with teachers and peers. Giving them access to the speech signal is only the first step toward developing an auditorily based spoken language system.

Setting appropriate expectations is critical if the full capacity of the device is to be attained. It is often difficult for teachers to expect the implanted child to depend on the auditory signal when the same expectation is not made for some of the other children in the class. On the positive side, all the students could improve their use of auditory input from the efforts made on behalf of the child with the implant. To prevent misinformation from being spread among peers, the teacher, parent, and/or child should explain to the class what the implant can and cannot do.

The percentage of implanted children in mainstream education settings has remained at a steady 35% level. The regular education teacher will continue to require in-service training regarding classroom modifications and realistic expectations. If the implant surgery occurs during the school year, the classroom teacher should receive information on the surgery, device, and expected performance.

Regardless of the educational setting, the student will require intensive individual therapy to improve his/her speech perception/production skills (Moog and Geers, 1991). Intervention takes into account the saliency of the acoustic features of speech, initially focusing on the higher-frequency vowels and consonants. The greatest impact on speech production occurs when the student is expected to repeat the stimuli and evaluate his/her own production. Especially critical is the transfer of newly acquired listening skills into real-life situations.

VIBROTACTILE SYSTEMS

Some children who cannot make use of traditional amplification because of the severity of their hearing loss may be candidates for a vibrotactile system. The commercially available systems were developed to code speech so that it can be presented in a tactile modality and enhance the reception of spoken language. Most units are body worn and have an environmental microphone that receives environmental and speech sounds. Noise reduction components are included in the units to assist in presenting a clearer speech signal. If these low-frequency sounds were not suppressed there would be constant stimulation of the skin and important sounds could not be discriminated. Power to the units is provided by rechargeable batteries.

Weisenberger (1989) described and classified the different devices according to the number of channels of stimulation provided. A vibrotactile system is shown in Figure 3.2. The systems can also be classified as vibratory or electrical. The former provide the signal through a transducer that vibrates and is worn on the arm or the sternum. The latter present electrocutaneous pulses to the abdomen that feel like vibrations.

Single-channel tactile aids stimulate the skin at one point with an amplitude-modulated (AM) signal that is based on an extraction of the amplitude envelope of the incoming acoustic waveform. Basic auditory detection tasks, including identification of environmental sounds, are facilitated by this type of unit. The ability to perform more refined auditory tasks, such as discriminating among phonemes, is not possible with the single-channel tactile units (Weisenberger, 1991).

Multichannel tactile devices were developed to provide the kind of information that would allow the user to discriminate frequency. By coding frequency information spatially, on different areas of the skin, better performance can be obtained on tasks like phoneme identification. Two-channel devices essentially divide the acoustic signal into low- and high-frequency regions and send it to two different transducers. The shift in the vibrotactile pattern from the low to high or high to low

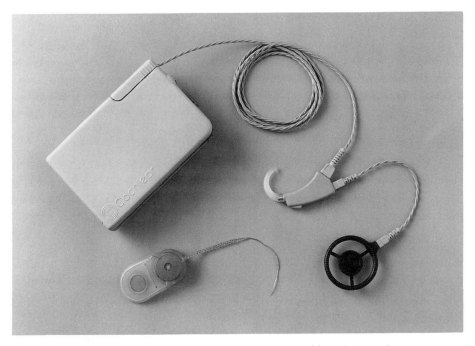

Figure 3.1a Cochlear implant transmitter provided by Cochlear Corporation, Englewood, CO.

transducer enhances the discrimination of the speech. Amplitude (loudness) changes are represented as changes in the intensity of the vibration. Aside from the improved discrimination ability, a two-channel device increases the ability to understand connected speech.

Increasing the number of channels (and the number of vibrators) to more than two significantly improves access to a greater portion of the frequency spectrum. The improvement in speech perception is even greater when speechreading cues are provided along with the tactile representation of the acoustic information. The consistency of the pattern of movement that results from changes in the stimulated transducers helps the child identify different phonemes in a word. However, more detailed information is provided (via a greater number of areas of stimulation) to represent duration, intensity, frication, and plosion. A higher number of channels allows for provision of other acoustic features of speech such as formants and their transitions (Lynch, Oller, and Eilers, 1989).

The auditory feedback loop that emerges so early in normally hearing children reflects the interdependence of speech perception and speech production. For the child using a vibrotactile system, feedback provides the comparison between his/her speech and the speech of others. The child tries to use his/her own speech to replicate the pattern he/she feels. In this way a tactile feedback loop is established (Eilers, Oller and Vergara, 1989).

There has been minimal research into the use of a tactile aid for speech perception and speech production. The few available studies demonstrate the benefit received from the use of the system with respect to speech production intelligibility (Weisenberger, 1989). A carefully designed training program that incorporates a tactile unit can also result in the successful speech and language development of young children who cannot benefit from traditional amplification (Eilers, Oller and Vergara, 1989).

Research is needed to determine the benefits of tactile aids for the profoundly hearing-impaired child. The greatest benefits demonstrated to date have been in the use of tactile devices to supplement receiving speech. Improved speech perception was found when a tactile device was added to speechreading, aided hearing, or a combination of the two, demonstrating the ability of children to integrate speech signals received through different modalities (Lynch, Oller and Eilers, 1989).

SOUND FIELD FM SYSTEMS

The individual FM systems described in Chapter 2 have become accepted devices for use in managing children in regular and special education settings. An individual unit is most appropriate for the child with bilateral permanent 30dB HL or greater sensorineural hearing loss. However, there are children (those with very mild or fluctuating hearing losses) for whom it is difficult to fit personal amplification, but who cannot cope with classroom listening conditions that interfere with the optimal reception of the speech signal. For those children, sound field FM systems, originally described in the early 1980s, may be of great benefit. A sound field FM system consists of a wireless FM microphone/transmitter that sends a signal to an integrated FM receiver/loudspeaker system (Sarff, 1981; Sarff, Ray, and Bagwell, 1981; Ray, 1989). By installing several (the number can vary from two to four depending upon room size) wall- or ceiling-mounted loudspeakers around the classroom space a positive speech-to-noise ratio is established (Flexer, 1991). As with the individual systems, the goal is to deliver a speech signal that is approximately 10dB louder than ambient room noise.

With this device, children continue to use their hearing aids, if prescribed, to monitor their own voices and those of the other children. The microphones of the hearing aids also receive the sound emanating from the loudspeaker. For the children who do not have personal amplification, the same relationship exists except that airborne amplified speech from the loudspeaker is received through the open ear. In either situation, the closer the children sit to the loudspeaker, the greater the intensity of the signal they receive; that is, the closer to the loudspeaker, the better the signal-to-noise ratio.

The rationale for sound field FM use is that regardless of the degree or type of hearing loss, the typical listening conditions in classrooms will interfere with the reception of the teacher's speech and therefore with access to information.

The number of children in regular education classrooms who can benefit from the sound field FM system is reported to be high. Flexer (1991) describes these children as having: (1) fluctuating hearing loss related to otitis media; (2) minimal sensorineural hearing loss with no personal amplification; (3) unilateral hearing loss, and (4) mild sensorineural hearing loss using personal amplification. A more complete description of these four groups of children is presented in Chapter 9. Flexer (1991) also points out the benefits of sound field systems for children with normal auditory sensitivity who demonstrate auditory processing problems.

As with any system, care must be taken to ensure its optimal function. Therefore, aside from troubleshooting the child's personal amplification, the microphone/transmitter of the sound field FM should be checked at the beginning of each school day to determine that the signal is at appropriate intensity levels.

ASSISTIVE DEVICES

Provision of amplification is basic to the management of individuals with hearing loss. However, there are circumstances in which even the most appropriate amplification will not result in the best access to a signal. Some of the devices depend on receiving an amplified signal via a remote microphone, while others provide the enhancement through a different modality, such as, writing. The need for providing a positive signal-to-noise ratio was presented in the discussion of FM systems (Chapter 2). Aside from those systems, there are numerous commercially available assistive devices that provide the hearing-impaired individual access to auditory signals through a variety of techniques ranging from television captioning to telephone amplifiers. The following is a discussion of assistive communication devices that may be appropriate for children with hearing impairment.

Use of a remote microphone (as with the individual FM system) is the most successful method of overcoming difficult listening conditions associated with high ambient noise levels and distance from the sound source. A large number of assistive listening devices capitalize on the strong signal created by placing a microphone at the sound source when that source is at a distance from the listener.

Large Group Listening Devices

With the individual wireless FM, the child wears a receiver and the speaker wears the microphone/transmitter. The speech is transmitted from the microphone on a

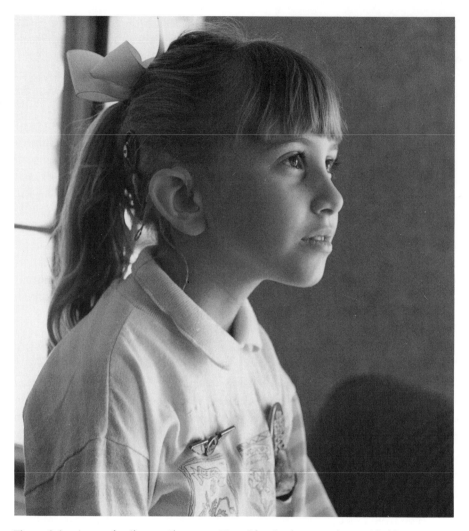

Figure 3.2 A sample vibrotactile sysem. Tactaid unit photograph provided by Audiological Engineering Corporation, Somerville, MA.

frequency-modulated (FM) signal, received by the child's unit, amplified, and delivered to the child's ear. Further, the receiver may be coupled through a snap-on transducer or the child's hearing aid via direct audio input or a teleloop (see Chapter 2). These systems can also be used when there are multiple listeners and one speaker. In that circumstance, the speaker uses one microphone/transmitter and the listeners all use receivers that are tuned to the same carrier frequency.

There are also listening devices that are installed in public facilities to accommodate large numbers of individuals with hearing loss. A common method of improving access to the auditory signal is the *induction loop system*, in which the speaker transmits over a microphone with the listener activating the telecoil in his/her hearing aid to couple to the induction loop. The signal is amplified in the receiver and a magnetic field is generated by a wire loop similar to the teleloop arrangement of a personal FM system coupled to the telecoil of the individual's hearing aid. The most obvious difference in this system is that the loop surrounds large areas, or even whole rooms (not just the person's neck), and may be permanent or temporary (Leavitt and Hodgson, 1984). As long as the individual is situated within the magnetic field of the loop and using a hearing aid with a good quality telecoil circuit, an audible, clear speech signal will be received.

Infrared systems also allow for reception in groups. The method of transmission is a carrier wave composed of an infrared light. Since it is a light signal, the system will work only in a single room (it cannot transmit through walls as a sound wave can) that does not let in sunlight. This type of system is most commonly found in large public places in which light is not critical, such as theatres (Wayner, 1986).

Other large group listening systems rely on a *hardwire* that physically connects the listener's hearing aid or headphones to the sound source. The source may be a microphone (for use in one-to-one communication), television, videocassette recorder (VCR), radio, or audiocassette.

Video Assistive Devices

For some hearing-impaired children, the audio channel of television or film is not loud or clear enough to be understood. For them, captioning is an invaluable assistive system.

Closed captioning provides a written transcript for the audiotrack of television programming. Individuals may purchase a captioning device that is used when a program emits a captioned signal. Since the promulgation of the American with Disabilities Act (ADA) in 1991, all televisions with a screen over thirteen inches will have captioning decoders built into them. *Open captioning*, which is seen by all viewers, is used for films and videotapes.

Real-time captioning provides a transcript for programming that is not prerecorded, such as news programs and interviews. These real-time devices require a trained stenographer, who types a verbatim transcript that is projected onto a television monitor or large screen for listeners who cannot hear all of the verbal information being presented.

Telephone Devices

The ability to use the telephone may be compromised for individuals with hearing loss. Various devices are available to increase access to the signal. The easiest accommodation for hearing aids is a *telephone amplifier*, which can be either attached to the handset or built into the telephone. The signal transmitted over the handset is amplified by 30% (Vaughn and Lightfoot, 1987). Some public telephones are equipped with amplifiers in the handset.

Some hearing aids have telecoil circuits that can receive an electromagnetic signal transmitted by the telephone. When the telephone switch is activated the microphone becomes inactive, leaving only the signal received through the telecoil. For individuals with mild to moderate hearing losses, telecoils are very beneficial. Greater degrees of loss may require the addition of amplifiers to access speech over the telephone (Flexer and Berg, 1990).

Another method of accessing the telephone signal for individuals who have greater degrees of hearing loss is the *TDD*. This device takes the spoken signal from the handset and converts it into a printed signal. The message can be seen on a small screen and/or produced in hardcopy. The most recent models of TDDs are portable and are available on some public phones.

Signaling and Alerting Devices

A number of *signaling and alerting devices* are available for the individual who cannot hear sounds such as the doorbell or telephone ringing or the baby crying. The method of signaling can be visual, as in lights flashing, or vibrotactile, as in an alarm clock. Some individuals choose a "hearing dog" to alert them to different sounds and auditory situations. As are guide dogs for the blind, these animals are permitted in public places.

A summary of the various assistive communication devices and their uses is presented in Table 3.1.

It is important to incorporate assistive communication devices into the life of a hearing-impaired child beginning at a young age. Including their use as part of auditory management programming establishes the devices as an integral part of the child's life. For example, parents can have a toddler use his/her hearing aid telephone switch to talk to a relative on the telephone in the same way a normally hearing child uses the phone. A teenager can be encouraged to babysit and make use of alerting devices when the baby cries. Television captioning is considered a potential source of learning for young hearing-impaired children. Reading skills may improve as a result of seeing the written word in programs viewed on a daily basis.

Continued changes in technology are expected to give greater access to auditory signals in all types of listening situations. For example, digital processing of signals has the potential to transmit information over telephone lines. Levitt (1991) reported on transmission of low-grade video pictures and text over conventional telephone lines, automatic speech recognition, and interactive video over cable television and conventional telephone lines. All of these devices could greatly increase the hearing-impaired individual's ability to use conventional systems.

Table 3.1   Assistive devices that may be beneficial to children (infant through school-age).

Device	Function	Purpose
Alerting: Doorbell Telephone Baby crying, etc.	Light flashes in a sequence on a board, a number of times. Hearing dog	Indicates that: Doorbell is ringing Telephone is ringing Baby is crying, etc.
Direct audio input: Television Radio Audio cassette	Hard wire connection from output of the electronic device to input of the amplification	Provides a positive S/N, amplifies the signal from the electronic device only for person using amplification
Telephone amplifier	Amplifies the acoustic signal from the telephone	Provides an amplified signal that can be heard with or without hearing aids
TDD*	Converts the acoustic signal from the telephone into a printed display	Provides access to the signal when it cannot be made loud enough with an amplifier or personal hearing aids
Closed captioning* *Open captioning* *Real-time captioning*	Presents a written text of the audio track across the bottom of the television screen	Provides access to the audio track of television programming when it cannot be heard with direct input or hearing aids

* The child must be able to read to make use of these devices. Captions are typically written at a fourth grade reading level.

SUMMARY

Advances in technology have significantly improved the lives of hearing-impaired people. Cochlear implants and vibrotactile systems have made the speech signal available to profoundly hearing-impaired children. Children with mild or fluctuating hearing losses have been accommodated by the sound field FM system, which establishes a positive signal-to-noise ratio in large group listening environments such as the classroom. Assistive devices can provide access to the world outside the child's home and school.

    Children and their families should be encouraged to begin using these systems early in the management process.

References

Eilers, R.E., Oller, D.K. & Vergara, K. (1989). Speech and language progress of hearing-impaired children in a systematic training program using tactual vocoders. In N.S. McGarr (Ed.) *Research on the Use of Sensory Aids for Hearing-Impaired People. Volta Review Monograph* 91:5, 127-138.

Flexer, C. (1991). FM classroom public address systems. Presentation at FM Auditory Training Systems Conference. New York, NY.

Flexer, C. & Berg, F.S. (1990). Beyond hearing aids: The mystical world of assistive communication devices. In C. Flexer, D. Wray, & R. Leavitt (Eds.) *How the Student with Hearing Loss Can Succeed in College: A Handbook for Students, Families and Professionals* (pp. 53-68). Washington, DC: A.G. Bell Association.

Koch, D., Seligman P., Daly, C. & Whitford, L. (1990). A multipeak feature extraction coding strategy for a multichannel cochlear implant. *Hearing Instruments* 41, 3.

Leavitt, R.J. & Hodgson, W.R. (1984). An effective home FM induction loop system. *Hearing Instruments* 5:47, 14-15.

Levitt, H. (1991). Recent research on innovative systems for telephone communication. Miniseminar presented at the annual Self-Help for Hard of Hearing People, Denver, CO.

Lynch, M.P., Oller, D.K. & Eilers, R.E. (1989). Portable tactile aids for speech perception. In N.S. McGarr (Ed.) *Research on the Use of Sensory Aids for Hearing-Impaired People. Volta Review Monograph* 91:5, 113-126.

Moog, J. & Geers, A. (1991). Educational management of children with cochlear implants. *American Annals of the Deaf* 136:2, 69-76.

Ray, (1989). Project MARRS—An update. *Educational Audiology Association Newsletter* 5:5, 4-5.

Sarff, L. (1981). An innovative use of free field amplification in regular classrooms. In R. Roeser & M.P. Downs (Eds.) *Auditory Disorders in School Children.* New York, NY: Thieme-Stratton.

Sarff, L.S., Ray, H. & Bagwell, C. (1981). Why not amplification in every classroom? *Hearing Aid Journal* 12,44-50.

Vaughn, G.R. & Lightfoot, R.K. (1987). ALD's pioneers: Past and present. *Hearing Instruments* 38, 4-6; 9-12.

Wayner, D.S. (1986). Assistive listening devices for improved communication and greater independence. *Hearing Instruments* 37, 21-24.

Weisenberger, J. (1989). Tactile aids for speech perception and production by hearing-impaired people. In N.S. McGarr (Ed.) *Research on the Use of Sensory Aids for Hearing-Impaired People. Volta Review Monograph* 91:5, 79-100.

4

Communication Modality

INTRODUCTION

The issue of communication modality selection has created enormous controversy in the field of deaf education. It is not the purpose of this chapter to promote one modality over another or to directly address the controversy. Rather, the three basic modalities will be described, considering family-related and education-related concerns.

An underlying principle of this chapter is that the vast majority (99%) of children, regardless of degree of hearing loss and/or communication modality, need optimal access to the speech signal. Spoken language must therefore be considered from the perspective of a child's needs in any communication system.

A great deal of controversy has long existed over the best system for a child with hearing loss to learn and use language. In an effort to circumvent that controversy, the traditional system names—oral/aural, total communication, cued speech, manual communication—will not be used in this chapter. Instead, the various systems will be described with respect to the way in which they enhance reception of spoken language. However, when referencing the work of others the formal names will be used.

Table 4.1 describes the input and output components according to system of communication. Use of hearing and speech is basic to all three systems listed. Hand gestures and formal signs are important as a means of adding cues to the spoken signal for the child who cannot completely rely on the use of hearing and/or the combination of audition and speechreading.

The professional involved in the initial decision must be aware that the choice of modality has a direct impact on all family members and will have ramifications for the setting in which the child will be educated. Families, the majority (92%) of which do not have additional members with hearing loss (Luetke-Stahlman and Luckner, 1991), must commit themselves to full-time use of the child's communication system. For example, even when a particular conversation does not include the child with hearing loss and speech is not directed to him/her, the use of the communication modality must be maintained. In this way the child with hearing loss will be able to "overhear" the conversation and acquire the various forms and content of language.

Table 4.1   Purpose: To improve the reception and production of spoken language.

Input/Output	Auditory	Speech	Sign/Cue
Auditory/Oral Auditory Verbal	x	x	
Cued Speech/Oral	x	x	x
Total Communication	x	x	x

Families in which English is not the primary spoken language must give special consideration to their choice of communicative modality. Questions will arise about the child's need to learn English—in spoken, written, or signed forms—if he/she is to attend regular education classes or programs for the hearing impaired.

Similar issues arise, particularly if the child does not have a hearing loss, when the parents and/or other siblings use American Sign Language (ASL), which is a non-English system, as the primary home language. However, the choice of a particular system is not always clear-cut, even in situations where the child has a profound hearing loss. The family's input is required and must be considered. For example, if deaf parents choose a total communication method, rather than ASL, they must consider the implications of that choice for their own language use. This is analogous to the hearing parents who chose a total communication method and must change their own interactive mode.

Regardless of the language and modality chosen, flexibility is critical. There may be situations in which a choice was initially made, and for a variety of reasons the child has not progressed as anticipated. In that case, the family and professionals must be willing and able to shift to a different method. The goal of intervention is to make the child linguistically competent.

Families may be strongly influenced by the audiologist who first diagnoses the hearing loss and attempts to predict the child's eventual communication skill development on the basis of an initial contact. It is clear that determining outcome from the degree of hearing loss by comparing data of students with equivalent hearing is a formidable, probably impossible task. In fact, professionals who categorize by hearing loss are guilty of making a self-fulfilling prophecy that may or may not be to the child's advantage. For example, the audiologist who feels strongly that all children with severe or profound hearing loss should be enrolled in a total communication program may be limiting the potential for some children to acquire spoken language competency. Conversely, the overzealous audiologist who believes that hearing, no matter how little, should be exploited in an effort to develop an auditorily based spoken language system, may be introducing a level of frustration intolerable to some children and families. Hearing loss, therefore, is just one factor to be considered when matching a family to a communication approach. Child, family, and community factors will all have an effect on the decision.

Child factors: hearing loss, age at onset, length of deafness, age, motivation, adjustment to amplification, intelligence, communicative skill development, social interaction, previous training.

Family factors: time, resources, commitment to an approach, adjustment to hearing loss, back-up support system, child management skills, home language, communicative demands of the home.

Community factors: availability of services, travel constraints, frequency of service.

These factors can be more important than the degree of hearing loss in determining the best match between the child, family, and program. What may be appropriate for the child with a positive profile on the child factors may not satisfy parental needs. Or child and parent factors may all be positive, but a program that meets their expressed objectives may not be available within a reasonable distance from their home. Depending on the family, this may or may not preclude their involvement in a particular kind of programming. Professionals in deaf education all can point to parents who with very minimal on site professional support have been able to assist their children in acquiring superior speech, language, or sign skills.

Two case histories exemplify the situation that faces the audiologist during the initial intake period. MD was identified as hearing impaired at seven months of age, but by nine months of age still had not received any amplification even though auditory oral programming had been recommended (Figure 4.1). A second opinion confirmed the results. The second center insisted that earmolds be made immediately and amplification loaned. This infant easily engaged adults in interactive communication through mutual eye gaze, gesture, and reciprocal vocalization. The mother insisted on teaching her child to speak even though, as a single parent, she had limited time, energy, and resources to devote to the habilitation process. A family support system was limited.

When the child, family and community factors are analyzed, it is clear that this child had the prerequisites to develop a functional spoken language system. However, family factors counteracted these effects, casting doubt on the end result.

Progress: This auditory-oral child is able to communicate with his mother, teacher, and classmates in simple phrases and sentences; however, his language level is significantly behind that of his hearing peers. At age four, he entered a self-contained class for hearing-impaired children in which the linguistic demands were somewhat reduced. He continues, at age six, to depend on speech as his major input and output mode.

AT, although first tested at fourteen months, was still being evaluated three months later. A second opinion at seventeen months confirmed the initial profound hearing loss and recommended immediate fitting of amplification (Figure 4.2). AT presented as highly noncommunicative at the initial evaluation. She rarely made eye contact with her conversational partner, relying instead on the adult's desire to fol-

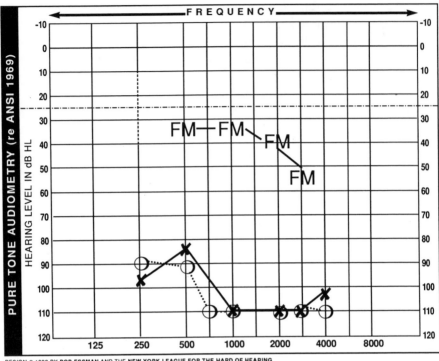

DESIGN © 1992 BY BOB ESSMAN AND THE NEW YORK LEAGUE FOR THE HARD OF HEARING

X left ear, unaided

O right ear, unaided

FM system

INITIAL DIAGNOSIS: 6 months
    Recommendation: Auditory/Oral
        No amplification after 2 months

SECOND OPINION: 8 months
    Recommendation: Auditory/Oral
        Immediate Amplification

FAMILY: Only child
    Single non-working parent

COMMUNICATION: Good voice quality
    Highly interactive
    Recognizeable vowels and consonants present

EXPECTATION: Strong commitment to only oral

Figure 4.1 Audiological, communicative, and family factors affecting program planning for child MD.

low her lead. Her vocalizations were either deep growls or high-pitched squeals, both of which provided kinesthetic feedback. AT's parents were unsure about what communicative modality to use with her. They decided to try an auditory-oral approach for a six-month trial period to determine if she was able to learn. As an only child of an intact family, AT had the advantage of the time and energy that the nonworking parent was able to give to the habilitation process.

In analyzing the child and family factors, it is apparent that the home environment was one in which language learning could occur. These parents were willing, eager, and committed to enhancing the language learning opportunities in the home. In contrast to MD, AT marginally met the criteria for inclusion in such a rigorous program.

Progress: Once amplification was loaned, many of the negative child factors dropped out. Notably, AT began to look at the speaker's face for clues to meaning as soon as she had some access to sound, and her vocalizations became more speech-like as she was able to monitor herself through hearing. At age six, she completed first grade in her home school with daily academic support and speech-language therapy. Her superior language skills place her in the top of her class compared to her normally hearing peers.

Given the initial status of these two children, it would have been difficult to predict the outcomes five years later. It is important to keep the other factors in mind when counselling parents regarding programming issues. Instead of dictating placement, the audiogram should be used to illuminate aspects of the speech signal potentially available to the child. A label should be used to categorize the degree of hearing loss, not the function of the person with the loss.

SUPPLEMENTARY SYSTEMS FOR ENHANCING RECEPTION OF LANGUAGE

The following section describes various systems that theoretically are used by individuals with hearing loss in order to access spoken language when hearing alone is insufficient. All of these systems require knowledge of spoken language because they are used in conjunction with English. This focus is consistent with the fact that 99% of school-age children with hearing loss use English, oral and/or signed, with only the remaining 1% using American Sign Language (ASL). More specifically, approximately one-third of children with severe and profound hearing loss use an oral/aural system, while the remaining two-thirds use a total communication system, and approximately 1% receive language through a Cued Speech modality (Woodward, Allen, and Schildroth, 1985). Since mild and moderate hearing loss is sixteen to thirty times more frequent than severe and profound, one can predict that a large number of children use an aural/oral mode of communication without any of these supplemental visual systems to receive spoken language. Considering these demographic data, it is clear that professionals working with hearing-impaired children need to

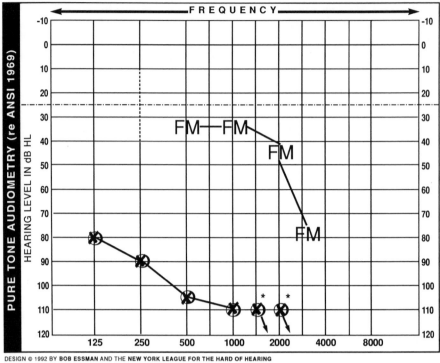

DESIGN © 1992 BY **BOB ESSMAN** AND THE **NEW YORK LEAGUE FOR THE HARD OF HEARING**

X left ear, unaided   **O** right ear, unaided   **FM**system   *No response

INITIAL DIAGNOSIS: 14 months
Recommendation: Total Communication
No amplification after three months

SECOND OPINION: 17 months
Recommendation: Auditory/Oral
Immediate amplification

FAMILY: Only child
Two parent family
One non-working parent

COMMUNICATION: Grunt-like sounds
Shrieks
Poor eye contact
Mouthing

EXPECTATION: Willing to use whatever modality the child needs

Figure 4.2   Audiological, communicative, and family factors affecting program planning for child AT.

be familiar with both the methods that maximize use of residual hearing, and those that supplement and enhance the auditory signal.

Speechreading Cues

The most common supplementary method for enhancing speech reception is speechreading. The visual saliency of speech sounds is dependent on a variety of factors that include the articulation of the sound and the environmental conditions of lighting and distance from and angle to the speaker (Jackson, 1988). Consonants are critical for discriminating among speech sounds. Auditorally there are many acoustic cues that can be used to discriminate among these phonemes. However, the same is not true for the visual cues. French-St. George and Stoker (1988) report on research indicating that only 25-30% of phonemes can be discriminated on a purely visual (facial) basis. Some consonants look the same on the lips (visemes) because they are made by the same movement of the articulators, e.g., /p/, /b/, /m/. Others cannot readily be seen because they are articulated in the back of the mouth, e.g., /k/, /g/. Therefore, the place of articulation (where the sound is made) of a consonant determines its visibility and thus its receptive intelligibility, with back consonants being less easily, visually discriminated (Erber, 1971). Further, discrimination errors tend to be made within the place of articulation category (Erber, 1974).

Early work in the receptive intelligibility of vowels indicated that a speechreader can visually discriminate among all the vowels (Nitchie, 1950). The greatest difficulty is in discriminating vowels that are adjacent to one another or in the same area of the vowel quadrilateral; that is, where they are produced in the mouth (Berger, 1972). Front and back vowels generally are not confused with each other and high and low vowels are not confused (Berger, 1970).

Coarticulation also affects the intelligibility of consonants. For example, Erber (1971) demonstrated that the vowel environment strongly influences consonant visibility, with open vowels providing the easiest speechreading condition.

Boothroyd (1988) explains that speechreading is highly dependent on knowledge of linguistic information. He describes the importance of the shared linguistic knowledge of the talker and the receiver that enables the receiver to depend on the constraints of the phonological and syntactic rules for correct perception. Boothroyd's data emphasizes the difficulty of relying on visual information alone.

In a review of the literature, Kaplan (1974) summarizes the problems associated with depending on speechreading as the sole source of cues for speech perception. They are as follows:

1. Visible movement clues make a decided contribution to recognition of consonant stimuli, particularly when little auditory information is available.

2. The distinction between voiced and voiceless cognates cannot be made when only visual clues are present.

3. Consonants produced in the front of the mouth are more visible and are identified correctly more frequently and more consistently than those produced farther back in the mouth.

4. According to some studies, consonant recognition seems to improve when the consonant is coarticulated with an open vowel. However, complete agreement does not exist on this point.

5. Consonant confusions tend to fall into viseme categories that are contrastive to each other but internally homophonous. However, there is little agreement as to the number or composition of those visemes which consist of nonlabial consonants. . .(pp. 21-22).

Gestural Cues

A method of providing visual cues to assist in discriminating spoken English phonemes was developed by Orin Cornett (1967, 1972). The method, which facilitates the acquisition of spoken language, uses handshapes and hand positions to supplement the information provided through speechreading. Cornett wanted to devise a system that would provide the profoundly deaf child with access to all of the sounds of speech, even when they cannot be heard. He argued that the limited visibility of speech sounds made reliance on speechreading cues alone quite inefficient.

By combining eight handshapes and four hand positions with speechreading, Cued Speech enables the receiver to discriminate among all the English phonemes. The four hand positions (base, larynx, chin, mouth) are used to indicate vowels that are grouped according to visual distinction. Vowels that cannot be visually discriminated are in different hand position groups; for example, /i/ is cued by a mouth hand position, while /I/ has a throat hand position cue. A diphthong combines the cues of the two vowels that make it, moving from the hand position of the initial vowel to that of the second vowel.

While the hand position is cueing the vowel, the handshape indicates the consonant group. The eight handshapes represent the groups into which the consonants have been divided on the basis of visible discrimination. As with the vowels, those consonants that look the same on the lips are in different cue groups. Thus, /p/ and /b/, produced with the lips together, have different handshapes, with /p/ being cued by extending only the index finger and /b/ cued by extending all fingers but not the thumb.

The Cued Speech system was designed to provide the young profoundly deaf child access to the entire speech signal through an alternative mode. Thus, he/she receives rich linguistic input and has the ability to acquire language in a natural way, like the child who uses hearing. Cornett (1975) also theorized that Cued Speech would improve a child's speechreading skills and help to develop the articulatory movements and vocalizations basic to intelligible speech production.

There is relatively little research data to either support or disprove Cornett's theory. That which supports Cornett can be summarized as follows:

1. Improvements in reception of spoken language varies greatly among school-age children using Cued Speech (Perier, Charlier, Hage and Alegria, 1990).
2. Reception of spoken language improves the most when Cued Speech is used in school and the home, slightly less when used only in the home, and much less when used only in school (Hage, Algeria and Perier, 1989).
3. Children using Cued Speech have a phonological equivalent that allows for identifying new words (Nichols, 1979).
4. There is a positive relationship between improvement through Cued Speech and a) degree of hearing loss, b) duration of exposure to Cued Speech, and c) age of initial exposure to Cued Speech (Hage et al., 1989).

Sign Systems

As indicated earlier, the majority of school-age children with severe and profound hearing loss use some mode of total communication; that is, communication in which speech, sign, and hearing are combined to expose the child to English. To enable these children to become competent in spoken and written English, manually coded English systems (for example, the Rochester method, Seeing Essential English, Signing Exact English, and Manual English) were developed.

Most of these systems incorporate aspects of ASL and English and are designed to be used in conjunction with speech. The grammar of English (e.g., word order) is maintained while some of the signs of ASL (e.g., nouns) and other modified signs are used. The difference among the systems relates to the development of the specific signs they use (Paul and Quigley, 1990).

When a manually coded English system is selected as the initial method of exposing a child to language, it is critical that the family become fluent as rapidly as possible in the combination of signs and speech. Care must be taken that the child's family and educational personnel are trained in the signs that are peculiar to the selected system. Obviously, serious problems will arise if different symbols are used in different settings. In some cases it is determined that an older child will benefit from the addition of signs to his/her use of auditory cues. At such times, it is critical that professionals and families understand that the child will have to be included in the training program. There is nothing about having a hearing impairment that provides a child with an inherent ability to know signs. The shift to a total communication system takes careful planning and may initially be slow.

For the child using a total communication system in a regular education setting, the use of a wireless FM system can be difficult. If an interpreter is used in the classroom, the child will have to decide to whom he/she should attend because the teacher will be providing the auditory input through the FM microphone/transmitter and the interpreter will be presenting the signs.

A thorough discussion of American Sign Language (ASL) is beyond the scope of both this chapter and book. It is a rule-governed language with its own semantics, syntax, phonology and pragmatic structure (Paul and Quigley, 1990). Accordingly, the information in this section does not apply to ASL and the management suggestions that follow would not be appropriate for children who use that language.

MAXIMIZING AUDITORY SKILLS

Regardless of the degree of hearing loss, a child's residual hearing should be maximally exploited for receiving the speech signal. This is true regardless of the communication system used.

Auditory Learning

Direct auditory intervention can be divided into several subgroups: (1) developing confidence in and dependence on listening; (2) training in the use of available acoustic cues; and (3) enhancing the listening-speaking connection. These primary areas of auditory learning can be targeted simultaneously in younger children and independently in older children.

Developing confidence in and dependence on listening
Dependence on hearing as a primary input mode is developed optimally from the first introduction of amplification (or other sensory device). If adults require the child to respond when auditory stimuli (speech or nonspeech) occur, then he/she can build on the information received through hearing, although it is an impaired input mode. Being dependent does not imply that the child is primarily auditory. Rather, it means that when visual clues are absent, as for example in darkened rooms, the child can use the auditory information received to decode some aspect of the message. The child best develops this confidence by spending time in situations in which the visual cues (speechreading) are eliminated or dramatically reduced. By carefully controlling the input according to linguistic complexity and familiarity and gradually increasing its difficulty, young children quickly learn to attempt new targets when introduced through the auditory channel. They learn that when aspects of the speech signal cannot be accessed through listening, the addition of speechreading cues can be used to fill in missing information.

For the older child with hearing loss who has the potential to depend on hearing for speech input but lacks the confidence to do so, the process is one of weaning from full visual access while simultaneously demonstrating the potential of accurately interpreting information received through the auditory channel. The structured, gradual reduction of visual speech cues coupled with success in hearing speech will make the child more confident and better able to rely on residual hearing.

Training in the use of available acoustic cues
Critical to the implementation of an auditory learning program is an analysis of the acoustic cues of speech that are available to the child when wearing amplification. If the primary frequency-specific cues fall within the child's aided residual hearing, then he/she should have access to them under optimal listening conditions. When misperceptions occur on these audible phonemes, the child is a candidate for specific practice, for example on pairs of words that demonstrate problematic contrasts. A complete description of a method for determining the audible of phonemes for the child using amplification and for planning a management program is presented in a following section.

Enhancing the listening-speaking connection
To strengthen the auditory-based feedback system for speech production, most children with hearing loss require practice in translating what they hear into intelligible speech. Younger children easily establish the auditory feedback loop since they have few habitual speech production patterns to overcome. If from the initiation of amplification children are required to repeat what they hear, then they have based their speech-sound categories on the comparison of what they produce and what they hear others produce. In this way they establish the ability to compare auditorily. Regardless of the age of the child and the difficulty that may be encountered, it is worthwhile to undertake this endeavor because of its benefits to speech production intelligibility. An awareness of the close connection between the auditory signal received and that produced orally is crucial for the child with hearing loss.

These general principles of auditory training are applicable to all children, regardless of their age or degree of hearing loss. The particular program and amount of direct service should be determined by careful evaluation of the child. It is particularly important that families and professionals be aware that the amplification device itself does not provide sufficient information for developing an appropriate auditory management program. Individually designed auditory management programs are especially important for children at either end of the hearing loss continuum, for whom appropriate programming is elusive.

Children with a mild or moderate hearing loss are typically the most misunderstood with respect to learning to use residual hearing. To assume that children with milder degrees of hearing loss understand and depend on the auditory signal for speech perception is erroneous. Often these children are "mismanaged" by empathetic, well-meaning professionals who "feel sorry" for these children who function on the perimeter of "normal." Instead of aggressively amplifying and rehabilitating children with mild and moderate hearing loss, they choose to minimize the potential difficulties in order to avoid calling attention to them. As adults, these children describe their anger at not receiving the same services and consideration as their more impaired peers. Yet it is the children with lesser degrees of hearing loss who represent the best investment for the school dollars spent on them. Too often services are not even considered for them because they can "get by" in many auditory situations. Little consideration is given to whether these children are living up to their potential levels of auditory, language, and academic performance (see Chapter 9).

At the other end of the continuum are those children in the profound hearing loss category, who also should not be excluded from developing maximum use of the auditory channel. Like those with mild hearing losses, these children are often not even considered candidates for auditory management. Despite the label "profound" and what it may signal to some professionals about a child's inability to use hearing, some members of this population can effectively use their residual hearing for speech reception. Without question, the degree of loss makes it doubtful that this subpopulation would become primary auditory learners without intensive training, but they certainly have sufficient access to speech to contribute equally with vision or to supplement what they receive through the visual channel. The challenge to the professional is to identify those children with auditory ability and exploit its full potential. For the remainder of the children in the profound hearing loss category, every effort should be made to gain as much benefit from audition as possible. The concept of total communication is dependent on this idea.

All children with hearing loss should be candidates for a strong program of auditory management. There is wide variability in the auditory skills of these children. The variability in performance given a similar hearing loss is for the most part attributable to the age of identification, amplification history, and previous training. Table 4.2 displays data that were collected on children with hearing loss who were being educated in the Connecticut public schools. These data demonstrate the serious error of relying on the audiogram to predict how well a child can use hearing for speech perception, and thus for learning language. The first two children (JV and MG) both have significant sensorineural hearing losses and are the same age. However, that is where the similarity ends. MG's language and academic performance are superior to those exhibited by JV. Further, MG's ability to use residual hearing is better than JV's, which is translated into greater speech production intelligibility. When the scores of TP are included, it is clear that even though he has better hearing, it is not possible to predict that he will perform better than a child with much poorer hearing (MG).

For children who cannot benefit from traditional amplification systems, access to the auditory signal is still possible. Cochlear implants, for example, give access to the speech signal at conversational speech intensity levels. However, it is only through intensive training that these profoundly deaf children can make functional use of the speech they receive. A complete discussion of sensory devices other than hearing aids and wireless FM systems, as well as candidacy for them, can be found in Chapter 3.

Table 4.2 Examples of hearing-impaired children for whom communication and academic performance cannot be predicted from degree of hearing loss.

Child	Degree of Loss	Age	Grade Placement	Language	Speech Intell.	Aud.Only Reception	Aud.-Vis. Reception
JV	bilateral severe to profound	14	one grade below (7th grade)	five years below age	fair	poor	fair
MG	bilateral severe to profound	14	on grade level (8th grade)	one year below age	good	poor	excellent
TP	bilateral moderate	14	one grade below (7th grade)	three years below age	good	good	good

Auditory Management

The following six auditory factors are critical to the success of any management program and are applicable regardless of the child's age or degree of hearing loss.

Daily troubleshooting of amplification

Functioning amplification is a prerequisite for implementing an auditory management program. Parents are responsible for checking the child's personal listening devices used in the home environment and school. It is particularly critical for the child learning language that the device be working at its best at all times. If problems arise they must be remedied immediately or loaner amplification should be acquired while the child's own is being repaired. Extended "down times" result in the child's missing important linguistic input.

When the child's personal and school-worn amplification are not the same device, it is the responsibility of school staff (as designated in the child's IEP) to trouble-shoot the equipment. There should be no assumptions that if the amplification was functioning properly before the child arrived at school that it will continue to do so for the entire day. It is particularly important that the troubleshooter check all components of a system, for example when the child's personal hearing aids are incorporated (through direct audio input or teleloop) into an FM system. School personnel should realize that monitoring the function of amplification is basic to ensuring that the child has optimal access to the teacher's speech and other classroom auditory information at all times. It is important that the personnel using the alternative sensory devices such as a cochlear implant, vibrotactile aid, sound field FM, and personal FM units are knowledgeable in the procedures for monitoring and making minor repairs. A more complete description of troubleshooting equipment and protocols can be found in the Appendix.

Modification of the listening environment

A child's listening environment varies significantly during the course of a day. Families and professionals must be aware of how dramatically the listening environment impacts on a child's ability to access the speech signal, and they must also be knowledgeable about methods of modifying the environment to improve these conditions. There must be careful analysis of the ambient noise levels, internal and external noise sources, and visual distractions, all of which can interfere with reception of the speech signal.

There are many methods for overcoming problems associated with the listening environment (Ross, Brackett, and Maxon, 1991). In brief, physical modifications such as carpeting the floor can reduce ambient noise levels and decrease reverberation, whereas the use of a wireless FM system can improve signal-to-noise ratios. Regardless of the method selected, improving the listening condition should be considered for all of the environments in which the child functions, both in home, day care, educational, and social settings.

Increasing the child's responsibility for amplification

The child must accept some responsibility for the care and maintenance of amplification or other sensory devices from the earliest stages. Before age two, this may take the form of reseating the earmold or indicating that the amplification is not functioning. Three-year-olds, if given the opportunity, can put on their own amplification and turn on the power. Changing the batteries must be monitored by an adult because of the danger of ingestion, but children should not be discouraged from participating in this activity. Independence in these early stages results in a school-age child who willingly uses and maintains amplification, reports problems, and can make some minor repairs.

A child who is mainstreamed must be able to independently manage his/her own equipment. This entails not only changing the batteries and performing some other aspects of troubleshooting, but also advocating appropriate use. Since it is difficult for the consultant to predict every situation that might occur during the school day, it is much more effective for the child to inform the teacher of the appropriate use of the FM microphone during the variety of classroom activities. The child who is adequately informed can act as his/her own advocate.

The same is true for the child who uses hearing aids rather than an FM system in the classroom. When the child is unable to hear the teacher, he/she should be allowed to improve the signal-to-noise ratio by moving closer to the primary sound source. The child who is knowledgeable about the proper use of amplification in a variety of listening conditions can function well in the regular education classroom without interfering with the usual classroom events.

Improving parents'/professionals' knowledge of the selection,
use, and maintenance of amplification
Successful amplification use is dependent on families and professionals understanding the rationale for the child-specific amplification recommendations. Their being
informed about the function of personal and school-worn amplification and/or other
sensory devices is also important to success. A complete description of the various
types of amplification and their maintenance can be found in Chapter 2 and that
related to other sensory devices in Chapter 3.

Increasing parents'/professionals' expectations for
auditory responses
Very young children spend most of their waking hours with parents (primary
caregivers) who must understand the importance of expecting and recognizing their
child's auditory responses. By establishing this expectation the parents begin to orchestrate opportunities for the child to respond through hearing rather than immediately relying on nonauditory stimuli. An initial important behavior is the manner
in which parents attempt to gain their child's attention. While calling the child's
name is the most natural method, most parents prior to diagnosis have resorted to
visual or tactile means of getting the child's attention, including tapping the child,
flashing lights, or stamping on the floor; their expectations for responses to auditory
signals are limited.

 Auditory expectations cannot be established without consistent use of amplification. Parents need to understand that without amplification their child is inca-
pable of receiving any of the rich verbal input surrounding him/her. If they realize
that critical moments are wasted when full-time amplification is delayed or inconsistent, they are more likely to insist on full-time use and expect auditory responses.
If there is a blasé attitude on the part of professionals, the parents will almost certainly adopt it. A consequence of increasing parental expectation is that the program
must have backup amplification equipment available to support the parents' con-
tention that "every minute counts."

 For the older child, nonauditory habits need to be broken. As the child becomes
better able to rely on amplified residual hearing, the home and classroom expectations must change to incorporate his/her changing abilities. As with any method of
behavior change, the demands and acceptances of the environment must accommodate and reinforce the increased abilities.

Providing information to extended family/professionals
Parents are often recipients of huge amounts of information on hearing loss and
amplification, either during counselling sessions with the audiologist or during par-
ent/infant communication training sessions. With grandparents, aunts, uncles, cous-
ins, and older siblings offering a much-needed respite to the family there is a need
to prepare them for managing the listening and learning needs of the child. Parents

who are committed to optimizing every daily routine and activity are much more comfortable leaving their child with these family members when they are sure that they understand the nature of the problem and appear competent to provide rich input. As the parents attempt to inform immediate or extended family, the information becomes second hand, filtered through the eyes of the parents. Thus, direct contact should be established with these family members by having them intermittently attend therapy sessions.

Information is also inefficiently conveyed in the educational environment. Too often information is given only to the child's case manager and no effort is made to provide in-service training to other school personnel. Obviously, the classroom teacher should know about the child's hearing loss, how amplification functions, and how the child performs with it. In addition, the negative effects of noise, reverberation, and distance from the sound source must be carefully explained. However, it is not only the classroom teacher who must have general knowledge about hearing loss and information specific to an individual child—any professional who provides direct service or comes in contact with the child during the school day should know how well the child can communicate, receptively and expressively. Since peers play an important role in the child's educational and social experience, specifically adapted in-service sessions can be effective for them as well (Maxon, 1990; Ross, Brackett, and Maxon, 1991).

Accessing the auditory signal

Basic to any auditory management program is an understanding of the acoustic components of the speech signal that normally hearing listeners use to correctly identify and discriminate speech sounds. Combinations of frequency, time, and intensity cues differentiate vowels and consonants according to voicing and manner features (time versus intensity) and place of articulation (time versus frequency). It should be noted that this review deals with static measures of speech acoustics without considering the constantly changing influence of the surrounding phonemic environment.

A great deal of linguistic information is carried by the suprasegmental components of speech. The speaker conveys stress, intonation, and rhythm by frequency and intensity changes. Most of those changes are carried on the fundamental frequency that falls below 300 Hz for all speakers (Peterson and Barney, 1952). Children with very minimal low-frequency hearing will have access to those suprasegmental patterns and will be able to learn to use the crucial linguistic information conveyed.

Vowels   Vowels produced in isolation can be discriminated by their relative formant patterns. During vowel production the complex sound generated at the vocal folds travels up the vocal tract, resonating in different regions. As the speaker changes configuration of the vocal tract, different areas of resonance, (formant frequencies) are produced. Table 4.3, developed from Peterson and Barney's data, represents the

Table 4.3   First and second formants (F1 and F2) of American English vowels spoken by males and females.

		|	|I|	|æ|	|ɔ|	|ʊ|	|u|	|ʌ|
		/i/	/I/	/æ/	/ɔ/	/ʊ/	/u/	/ʌ/
F1 (Hz)	Male	270	390	660	570	440	300	640
	Female	310	430	860	590	470	370	760
F2 (Hz)	Male	2290	1990	1720	840	1020	870	1190
	Female	2790	2480	2050	920	1160	950	1400
F2/F1	Male	8.48	5.10	2.61	1.47	2.32	2.90	1.86
	Female	9.00	5.77	2.38	1.56	2.47	2.57	1.84

Adapted from Levitt (1978). Data from Peterson and Barney (1952).

first two formants (F1, F2) of the various English vowels spoken by a male and female. The concomitant changes of the vocal tract and formant frequencies for each of the vowels can also be seen. For example, the back vowel /ɔ/ has F1 and F2 values that are close, while F1 and F2 of the front vowel /i/ are separated by a much greater distance. The distance between F1 and F2, the relative formant frequency relationship, is used for between-vowel discrimination.

It is important to note that the relative formant frequency values rather than the absolute values are used. Table 4.3 shows that although absolute frequencies differ across speaker groups, the relative difference between F1 and F2 (formant ratio) remain fairly constant. For example, the range of the formant ratios for the vowel /i/ is 8.48 (men) and 9.00 (women). However, the formant ratios for different vowels vary in the same manner regardless of speaker, e.g., 9.00 for /i/ versus 2.57 for /u/ (Levitt, 1978).

The information in Table 4.3 can be used to understand that children with hearing loss should be able to hear much of the formant information. Even those whose residual hearing is limited to the frequency region below 1000 Hz will have access to the F1 of all of the vowels. In order to gain all of the vowel information provided by the formant ratios, the child would need to have hearing through 3000 Hz.

Consonants   The acoustic cues used to identify consonants are considerably more complex. The English consonants are divided by the distinctive features of voicing, manner, and place of articulation (Table 4.4).

Voicing is carried by several different cues, one of which is voice onset time (VOT)—the relationship of the time at which the vocal folds begin to vibrate compared to the release of the articulators. When they begin at the same time, the con-

Table 4.4 Consonants of English categorized according to the distinctive features of voicing, manner, and place of articulation.

| | | | VOICING | | | PLACE | | | |
			Bilab.	Labiodent.	Lingdent.	Alveolar	Palatal	Velar	Glottal
	Plosive	Unv	p			t		k	
		V	b			d		g	
	Fricative	Unv		f	th	s	sh		h
		V		v	TH	z	^		
M A N N E R	Nasal	V	m			n		n^	
	Semivowels	V	w					j	
	Liquids	V				l, r			
	Affricates	Unv					tsh		
		V					d^		

sonant is voiced, while longer VOTs occur in voiceless consonants. Another voicing cue is the duration of an adjacent vowel. The same vowel will differ in duration according to the voicing of the consonant environment, e.g., /I/ is shorter in "picks" as compared to "pigs." Voicing cues fall in the lower frequency range (≤300 Hz).

A stop can be identified by (1) silence during articulator occlusion; (2) the burst of energy corresponding to articulator release; and (3) the direction and degree of F2 transition. Voicing of stops and nasality causes different types of acoustic energy surrounding and/or preceding the transitions.

The presence of low-frequency energy (around 300 Hz) of fairly long duration is an indication that the consonant is a nasal. The presence of antiformants, i.e., regions of acoustic energy where harmonics of speech are suppressed, occurs above 3000 Hz and in areas adjacent to F2 for nasal consonants.

Fricatives are longer in duration than stops; for example, /s/ is longer than /t/. Fricatives as a group share similar frequency characteristics, but place of articulation affects the frequency range of the hiss produced by the airstream being forced through the closely approximated articulators. Those frequency bands are /f/ = 1500-7500 Hz, /s/ = 3500-8500 Hz with a 4200 Hz peak, /sh/ = 1600-7000 Hz band with 2200, 2800, 4000 Hz peaks, and /th·/ = 1400-8000 Hz. The voiced cognates have additional low-frequency information around the fundamental frequency.

Although beyond the scope of this chapter, the reader should be aware that coarticulation is critical during ongoing speech. For example, vowel interaction with consonantal effects can change the direction and degree of the F2 transition. Although the child may be unable to hear the actual consonant that ends the word, he/she may be able to hear the direction and duration of the transition, which provide clues to identifying the final sound. For example, even when the final consonants of "cat", "cab", "cad", and "cam" are not audible, it is possible for a listener to identify which word was said without watching the face.

The child with congenital hearing loss has access to many fewer consonant cues than does the child with normal hearing; however, the redundancy of the cues makes it unnecessary to always use them all. The purpose of the model is to provide the professional with an awareness of the relatively large number of cues that are available to a particular child and how well he/she uses them.

The careful analysis of the model is important because an error that appears unreasonable to the individual with normal hearing may be understandable when considering the reduced acoustic cues available to the hearing-impaired person. The following example, confusing /i/ and /u/, can readily be explained by the acoustic cues. The vowel /i/ has a very low F1 (270 Hz) with a high F2 (2290 Hz). The vowel /u/ also has a low F1 (330 Hz), but a relatively low F2 (870 Hz). When the acoustic information is considered, the child with a high-frequency hearing loss whose amplification does not provide sufficient high-frequency aided hearing will not receive the second formant of /i/. Therefore it will be difficult to decide whether he/she heard /i/ or /u/.

Although this book does not deal with the assessment process that must precede any appropriate management program, a brief discussion of it is necessary. It is included here because, although presented at conferences, it does not appear in print. The technique of plotting speech acoustic information on an aided audiogram can be used to determine the specific speech sounds that are available to a particular child. This procedure is basic to planning auditory management.

Boothroyd's (1984) isophonemic word lists, which were developed to be scored on a phoneme-by-phoneme basis, are presented to the child at a normal conversational level (45-50dB HL, or an estimate by the clinician) with no visual cues. The child is instructed to repeat exactly what was heard, regardless of whether it sounds like a word, and the phonetic transcription is recorded for each stimulus. The analysis is accomplished by plotting the primary acoustic cues of the stimulus and the child's response, and plotting those frequency and intensity relationships on the aided audiogram (Maxon, 1982).

The next step in the procedure is to compare the child's response, phoneme by phoneme, to the stimulus item, and then to the aided warble tone audiogram. Table 4.5 displays the frequency bands of acoustic energy for the consonants. Intensity of those bands, in dB HL, is seen in the right-hand column. Although these mean values are static and do not represent running speech, they are considered representative

Table 4.5   Consonant frequency bands as a function of intensity.

| Consonant | Frequency Bands | | | | Intensity |
	1	2	3	4	(dB HL)
/r/	600-800	1000-1500	1800-2400		46
/l/	250-400		2000-3000		45
/sh/			1500-2000	4500-5500	41
/ng/	250-400	1000-1500	2000-3000		41
/t/			1500-2000	4000-5000	38
/n/	250-350	1000-1500	2000-3000		37
/j/	200-300		2000-3000		36
/m/	250-350	1000-1500	2500-3500		35
/thᵛ/	250-350			4500-6000	34
/t/			2500-3500		34
/k/			2000-2500		34
/f/				4000-5000	34
/g/	200-300		1500-2500		33
/h/			1500-2000		32
/s/				5000-6000	32
/z/	200-300			4000-5000	31
/v/	300-400			3500-4500	31
/p/			1500-2000		30
/d/	300-400		2500-3000		29
/b/	300-400		2000-2500		29
/th⁻/				6000	28

and are workable estimates of the sounds. To facilitate the analysis, the frequency and intensity cues can then be superimposed on the aided audiogram, and a comparison made between the stimulus phoneme and the response error phoneme.

Figure 4.3 displays the hearing of a child who made several errors on the words lists.

The acoustic cues for /dz/ and /z/ are shown below.

Phoneme	Primary frequency bands		Intensity
/dz/	200-300 Hz	2000-3000 Hz	36 dB HL
final sound in page			

| /z/ | 200-300 | 4000-6000 Hz | 34 dB HL |
| final sound in pays | | | |

When the energy for /dz/ is displayed as the crosshatched rectangles and the energy for /z/ as the solid rectangles, the low-frequency bands (200-300 Hz) for both

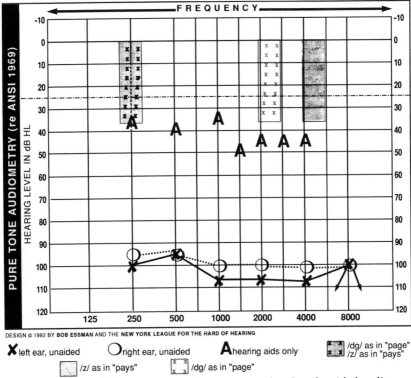

Figure 4.3 Analysis of phoneme perception errors as related to the aided audiogram.

phonemes overlap while the high-frequency bands do not. Since this child's aided residual hearing does not allow the high-frequency energy to be audible while at least part of the low-frequency information is, this error that maintains the voicing feature is considered reasonable. That is, this child uses the low-frequency voicing cue, but cannot hear the higher frequency bands of energy that could be used to distinguish between the two phonemes.

If the same child had better high-frequency hearing or amplification that provided more high-frequency gain, more of the acoustic information would be available and the perceptual error might not occur.

SPEECH/LANGUAGE ACQUISITION

In Table 4.1 all the modalities include the auditory channel as an input mode and speech as an output mode. Whether these are the primary means of receiving and producing speech or are used in conjunction with other modes depends on the parents' choice.

The development of functional speech skills requires much more than requiring just that the child use voice. It takes the concerted effort of the child, parent, and school to refine the gross vocalizations into recognizable words and phrases. For the child who is using speech as his/her primary expressive mode, the need to achieve a high level of intelligibility is urgent and motivating. For those students who have additional expressive modes, there is less immediate need to validate the effort required.

The development of speech proceeds through a sequence of steps that can be facilitated through appropriately targeted intervention. The infant learns to produce the entire repertoire of speech sounds through a process of internal feedback and external reinforcement. The infant produces random vocalizations that adults interpret according to the situational context and the resemblance of the vocalization to real words.

The speech sound repertoire of newly-identified hearing-impaired infants is necessarily limited by their reliance on tactile/kinesthetic feedback for self-monitoring. When amplification is fitted, an auditory-feedback system becomes a viable alternative. To activate this auditory-feedback system, the infant needs to compare his/her production sounds to the models heard every day. For children with severe and profound hearing losses and those with cochlear implants, this will happen only through the concerted effort of educators and parents. Since such children do not overhear the speech of others, their exposure to the rich verbal examples of their environment is limited. Parents need to increase their infants' access to the comparative models by increasing the amount and clarity of input presented at close range. Educators must expect and insist on "best" productions during school hours.

Refinement of the speech system is accomplished through systematic steps that are engineered by rehabilitation providers, teachers, and family. The targets should be developmentally appropriate and relevant to the speech needs of the student. The speech targets should be chosen according to the normal developmental sequence, the acoustic characteristics of the phoneme, and the ability of the child to produce the prerequisite features or other phonemes in the family of sounds.

For the young hearing-impaired child, focusing on phonemes that are late-developing in the normal population is asking for failure. Early developing sounds should be addressed first as long as the acoustic characteristics of the phoneme places the cues within the child's aided residual hearing. Fortunately, normally hearing infants begin with the vowels, which have acoustic energy in the region audible to almost all hearing-impaired children. Development progresses to the most advanced phonemes, which require much more coordinated movement of the articulators to formulate correct production, such as the /tsh, dth⁺,/ and the fricatives /s,sh/.

Next, teaching/stimulation techniques that achieve the correct production and use of the sound must be developed. Although imitation plays a role in the initial shaping of the phoneme, it has limited usefulness when the child is learning to use and monitor the sound. Therefore, as soon as the correct approximation has occurred the child should be accountable for retrieving the production on his/her own. The final step is to reduce all external cues, making the student totally responsible for remembering how and when to use the phoneme. The need to use functional words or phrases as the stimuli that occur frequently in a variety of situational contexts is critical to the success of speech production training.

The third factor to be considered is the need to facilitate generalization of newly learned skills. Often professionals and parents expect the student to immediately use the new phoneme in all contexts once correct production is achieved in isolation. There are many more steps to the process, including the requirement that the child self-monitor his/her own productions within the structured environment of the remedial sessions. Carryover occurs when children can determine whether their production is correct and modify it if necessary. Automatic use is just a short step from this self-correction phase.

SUMMARY

Communication development can follow a variety of paths when an infant is hearing impaired. Maximizing use of residual hearing through the use of amplification or other sensory aids facilitates acquisition of English, other spoken languages, and their symbolic representations. The particular method of communication a child uses is dependent on a variety of factors that incorporate the needs of the child, family, and community. Regardless of the method, intervention should begin as soon as the hearing loss is identified and amplification provided.

References

Berger, K.W. (1970). Vowel confusions in speechreading. *Ohio Journal of Speech and Hearing Monograph 5,* 2.

Berger, K.W. (1972). *Speechreading: Principles and Methods.* Baltimore, MD: National Education Press.

Boothroyd, A. (1984). Auditory perception of speech contrasts by subjects with sensorineural hearing loss. *Journal of Speech and Hearing Research, 27,* 134-144.

Boothroyd, A. (1988). *Hearing Impairment in Young Children,* Washington, DC: A.G. Bell Association.

Cornett, R.O. (1967). Cued Speech. *American Annals of the Deaf* 112, 3-13.

Cornett, R.O. (1972). Cued Speech. In G. Fant (Ed.) *International Symposium on Speech Communication Ability and Profound Deafness.* Washington, DC. A.G. Bell Association.

Cornett, R.O. (1975). Cued Speech and oralism: An analysis. *Audiology and Hearing Education* 1, 26-33.

Erber, N.P. (1971). Effects of distance on the visual reception of speech. *Journal of Speech and Hearing Research* 14, 848-857.

Erber, N.P. (1974). Visual perception of speech by deaf children: Recent developments and continuing need. *Journal of Speech and Hearing Research*, 178-185.

French-St. George, M. & Stoker, R. (1988). Speechreading: An historical perspective. In C.L. DeFilippo & D.G. Sims (Eds.) *New Reflections in Speechreading. The Volta Review Monograph* 90:5, 17-31.

Hage, C., Algeria, J. & Perier, O. (1989). Cued Speech and language acquisition. Paper presented at the Second International Symposium on Cognition, Education and Deafness, Washington, DC.

Jackson, P. (1988). The theoretical minimal unit for visual speech perception: Visemes and coarticulation. In C.L. DeFilippo & D.G. Sims (Eds.) *New Reflections in Speechreading, The Volta Review Monograph* 90:5, 99-115.

Kaplan, H. (1974). The effects of Cued Speech on the speechreading ability of the deaf. Unpublished doctoral dissertation, College Park, MD: University of Maryland.

Levitt, H. (1978). The acoustics of speech production. In M. Ross & T.G. Giolas (Eds.) *Auditory Management of Hearing-Impaired Children* (pp. 45-116). Baltimore, MD: University Park Press.

Luetke-Stahlman, B. & Luckner, J. (1991). *Effectively Educating Students with Hearing Impairments*. White Plains, NY: Longman Publishing Group.

Maxon, A.B. (1982). Speech acoustics: A model for managing hearing-impaired children. Presentation at the American Speech-Language-Hearing Association Conference, Toronto, Canada.

Maxon, A.B. (1990). Implementing an in-service training program. In M. Ross (Ed.) *Hearing-Impaired Children in the Mainstream*. Parkton, MD: York Press.

Nichols, G.H. (1979). Cued Speech and the reception of spoken language. Unpublished Master's thesis, Montreal, Canada: McGill University.

Nitchie, E.B. (1950). *New Lessons in Lipreading*. Philadelphia, PA: Lippincott Co.

Paul, P.V. & Quigley, S.P. (1990). *Education and Deafness*. White Plains, NY: Longman Publishers.

Perier, O., Charlier, B., Hage, C. & Algeria, J. (1990). Evaluation of the effects of prolonged cued speech practice upon reception of spoken language. *Cued Speech Journal* 4, 47-59.

Peterson, G.E. & Barney, H.L. (1952). Control methods used in a study of the vowels. *Journal of the Acoustical Society of America,* 39, 151-168.

Ross, M., Brackett, D. & Maxon, A.B. (1991). *Assessment and Management of Mainstreamed Hearing-Impaired Children: Principles and Practices*. Austin, TX: Pro-Ed.

Woodward, J., Allen, J. & Schildroth, A. (1985). Teachers and deaf students: An ethnography of classroom communication. In S. Delancey & R. Tomlin (Eds.) *Proceedings of the first annual meeting of the Pacific Linguistics Conference* (pp. 470-493). Eugene, OR: University of Oregon.

5

Programming:
Infants and Toddlers

INTRODUCTION

Hearing impairment of even the mildest degree can result in long lasting communicative, social, and academic deficits. Public Law 99-457 mandates that each participating state provide services to its infants and toddlers that are at risk for educational delay, as well as to their families. Under its terms, service providers must develop an Individualized Family Service Plan (IFSP) to address the delays evidenced by the infant during multidisciplinary evaluations. Recognizing the importance of parents during these early years, the federal government stressed that intervention must include not only the services that the infant requires, but also those needed by the family to provide a stimulating, growth-enhancing environment.

The portions of the IFSP unique to the hearing-impaired infant are listed in Table 5.1. In addition to the auditory/communicative considerations presented, information should be included on the infant's development in nonhearing-related areas (e.g., fine motor, gross motor, cognitive).

PARENT EDUCATION

The role of professionals in managing hearing-impaired children is clearly defined. The parents however, are often the forgotten team member. Parents provide a continuity to the child's education that cannot be achieved by professionals, who often change from year to year. Parental involvement that directly impacts on the auditory, communicative, academic, and social needs of the hearing-impaired infant continues to impact indirectly during the remainder of the child's life, including the school years.

Parent/Child Interaction

Soon after their child is born, all parents identify strategies that are effective in engaging him/her in communicative exchanges. At the earliest stages, these routines

Table 5.1   Listing of the communicative assessments and management unique to the Individualized Family Service Plan of the prelingually deaf infant.

I. Assessing the Communicative Skills of the Hearing-impaired Infant
    -receptive modality
        audition
        visual
        combined visual and auditory
        gesture
        in noise and distance conditions
        parental expectations
    -comprehension
        of situation
        of gesture
        of word/sound associations
        of words
        of word combination
        of phrase/sentence
    -production
        of gesture
        of word/sound associations
        of word
        of word combination
        of phrase/sentence
    -expressive modality
        speech
            vocalization
            babbling
            sound repertoire
        gesture
            general/nonspecific
            specific/meaningful
        facial expression
        eye gaze
    -parent/child interaction
        engagement style
        selection of activity
        analysis of child's level of interest
        attention-getting
        loudness level
        adaptation to the child's language level

II. Designing an IFSP from Evaluation Data
    -communicative areas for intervention
        use of audition
        comprehension and production of spoken language
        speech production
        use of language
        parent/child interaction
    -place of implementation
        home
        intervention/therapy program
    -person responsible
        professional
        parent
    -equipment required
        FM unit
        hearing aids
    -frequency of service based on:
        degree of hearing loss
        age at identification
        use of amplification
        age entering intervention program
        parental involvement
        other handicapping conditions

Table 5.2 Parents' role in managing the auditory, communicative, academic, and social needs of the hearing-impaired child.

1. AUDITORY

Direct: recognition of the loss
control of hearing aid use
troubleshooting amplification equipment
monitoring of the listening environment in nursery school and
    at home
arranging and keeping appointments

Indirect: help gain independence in monitoring the equipment
advocate for hearing in school
explain amplification to school personnel

2. COMMUNICATION

Direct: facilitate acquisition of language through quality input

Indirect: refine in a naturalistic way
understand relation to academic
provide experiences relative to vocabulary
review vocabulary of lessons
provide reinforcement

3. ACADEMIC

Direct: prepare child for nursery school concepts and vocabulary
liaison with teacher and therapist
reinforce classroom language

Indirect: help do homework
provide related experiences
assist in carryover

4. SOCIAL

Direct: orchestrate opportunities for social interaction
provide appropriate social language in context
normal behavioral models

Indirect: fine-tune skills
provide models for social language
teach child the consequence of actions
instruction in sex education

consist of exaggerated facial expression, eye-widening, eyebrow lifting, and head movement combined with vocalizations that vary widely in intonation contour. The visual aspects of these interaction strategies cause the child to react by smiling, establishing eye contact, and/or vocalizing. Since the infant's vocalizations are reflexive or vegetative in the early months and therefore less dependent on hearing, it is not surprising that normally hearing and hearing-impaired infants respond equally well to their parents' overtures.

Between four and six months, there is a change in the kind and use of the infant's vocalization due to the emergence of an auditory-feedback loop. It is during this period that the child's vegetative/reflexive vocalizations diminish in favor of more intentional, auditorily monitored and propagated babbling. The parents of normally hearing infants begin to elicit reciprocal vocal responses as they continue their visual/nonverbal exchanges. However, hearing-impaired infants are unable to use hearing to monitor their own and others' vocalizations. Their vocalizations thus stay at the rudimentary level established during the earlier period and only on rare occasions become reciprocal. Nonvocal engagement techniques continue to be effective in maintaining the hearing-impaired child's interest as long as visual attention is initially obtained. At this relatively early stage, parents may be unaware that they have already changed their style to include more of the visual aspects of the interactive signal.

Between six and twelve months, children with normal hearing refine their communication to include long strings of reduplicated babbling used to express a variety of intents that are easily discernible to the parents. Although parents continue to use highly exaggerated intonation to obtain and maintain the child's attention to salient words and phrases, they rely less on the visual attention-getters and engagers. It is at this point that the differences in the interaction styles of the two groups of parents becomes most apparent. The parents of hearing-impaired children maintain highly visual engagement strategies while the parents of normally hearing children have adopted a more auditorily based verbal interaction style.

It is the combination of parent intent and child feedback that determine the course of interaction between the partners. It is therefore not unusual for hearing-impaired children, identified between the ages of one and two years, to be functioning in a communicative environment that reflects their own visual dependence. Over time, the child has shaped parental input to meet his/her particular underdeveloped communication status. It would be unusual for parents to be totally unresponsive to their child's feedback.

Most parents are unaware of the extent to which they have modified their speech input so that their child can understand them. Typically they use simplified syntax accompanied by context and gesture. These modifications emerge after months of identifying the most efficient means of transferring information and signal a responsive parent. However, for progress to occur, once the child has access to sound, the parent will need to have direct instruction in how to create an interactive atmosphere that is conducive to forward language learning.

Parents play a primary role in teaching language to their young hearing-impaired children. The process, constantly evolving, is one in which a change in the communication habits of one partner dramatically affects the communication habits of the other. As the child learns language, parents must constantly change the complexity of their language input to help him/her learn more advanced vocabulary and grammar. A mismatch between the child's needs and parental input results in the child's slow progress. Helping the parent make adjustments in the quality and quantity of parent language is one of the major goals of the communication training program.

A mismatch between parent and child is most noticeable in a natural language learning situation. Simulating a home environment in the clinical setting permits problematic behaviors to emerge and be addressed immediately by the therapist. Techniques such as helping the parent select more advanced vocabulary or more complex sentence structure to make a standard request have proven effective over time. For example, "Open the door" becomes "Let's see what is inside the cabinet." As the parents observe growth in the child's language, their use of more advanced input is reinforced. As a result of this "fine-tuning" process, the child makes more rapid progress over a shorter period of time.

Analysis of Parent/Child Interaction

An integral part of any diagnostic/therapeutic intervention with hearing-impaired infants is an analysis of the quantity and quality of parent-child communicative interaction. Parent report and direct observation provide the vehicles for analyzing parental input and child response.

Parent Report
A detailed communicative history is needed to corroborate the behaviors noted during the observation and to determine the quality of parental observation skills. The starting point should be a parental description of the child's skill level. The second step is to elicit the parents' estimation of their child's abilities relative to peers or siblings at that same age. Follow-up questions explore the behaviors that the child uses during specific daily routines, such as requesting to go outside, requesting food, refusing to comply with a request, calling a family member, etc. The cumulative information acquired should provide a detailed description of the child as perceived by the parents.

Observation
The parent and child are best observed during natural interaction in the home. Since they cannot usually be seen there, the examiner must orchestrate conditions that will

Table 5.3   Specific parent/child interaction factors to be observed.

Parent	Child
attention-getters	attention-getters
adapting to the child's interest	language level
complexity of parental input	eye contact
relative to the child's language	following nonverbal signals
equality of conversational turns	establish topic nonverbally
loudness	learning style
clarity	intents expressed
exaggerated intonation contour	responsiveness to parent's overtures
initiation/respondent ratio	
attention maintainers	
use of gesture	
use of visible explanations	
responsiveness to child's overtures	

elicit natural interactions within the unfamiliar school or agency setting. The parent and child should be placed in a comfortable room with age-appropriate toys. If parents believe that the purpose of the observation is to display the child's skills, they are more likely to naturally exhibit their own commonly-used elicitation and stimulation techniques.

Cole and St. Clair-Stokes, (1986) describe a videotape analysis for documenting the parent/child interaction factors that promote listening and spoken language in hearing-impaired children. Having a method of focusing the observation of the parent/child dyad assists the professional in enhancing the interaction and monitoring the changes that the parents effect. Table 5.3 describes the interactive behaviors pertinent to a conversational analysis.

Issues

Bilingualism

Because of the occurrence of hearing impairment across racial and ethnic boundaries, it is not unusual for a professional to be faced with a parent/child unit in which the home language is other than English. This situation poses several dilemmas. Parents, as the primary source of language stimulation, need to feel comfortable expressing the early developing forms in their native language. Even parents who have facility in English are more likely to resort to their "home language" for expression of these functional words and phrases. Even if the parents decide to use only English with the hearing-impaired infant, much of their other language use in the home will be non-English, for example during adult conversations or with normally hearing siblings. Thus the child has no opportunity to learn from the adult-to-adult or adult-to-other-child interactions.

The situation is complicated by the fact that the professional involved is unlikely to be fluent in the family's language. This individual cannot then provide the direct modelling and instruction needed for effective parent/child programming to occur. If, in the best of all situations, the professional and parents speak the same language, intervention is still compromised because the child is not learning the language in which he/she will be educated. It is the rare special education program that educates students in their home language, gradually introducing English as a second language. Therefore, children who have gained functional facility in their "home language" will still enter the structured school setting at a disadvantage. Although knowledge of one language can facilitate the learning of another, it is doubtful that by the age of three the hearing-impaired child will have sufficient linguistic sophistication to undertake such a task. Even single-language learning is difficult for the severely and profoundly hearing-impaired infant. Therefore, language learning in a bilingual environment is confounded because the child must learn that the same object/concept is represented by two different sounding words.

In an attempt to avoid the negative impact of learning two languages some bilingual parents take the extreme position of forbidding any use of "foreign" words around their hearing-impaired infant. As a result the child is left out of the rich ethnic or cultural community of which the family is a part. Although it is important to understand the complexities of the bilingualism, it is also critical to prepare children for inclusion in their community. A more moderate approach would be to use "foreign" words and phrases that have accepted usage within English sentences. For example, "tush" for buttocks, "tati", "papa", "papi", "abba", for daddy; or "ima", "meme", "mama" for mommy. Ethnic or cultural songs, prayers, and poems can all be learned in their original language, as long as the same material is not being presented simultaneously in English. It is the dual coding of the same act, object, or event that causes language learning to proceed slowly.

Cultural Diversity

Parent/child interaction can be affected by widely differing child-rearing practices based on ethnic and cultural group norms. Extended infantile behavior is accepted by many cultures, resulting in lowered expectations or decreased conformity to adult demands. Parents in these groups are less likely to view their child's communicative behavior as widely variant from the norm even when to the observer it appears to be so. Such parents often have difficulty identifying the communicative areas that need to be addressed in a management program, and little progress is made because parental commitment to the goals and objectives of the program is minimal. Other cross-cultural variations include a parent-child interaction style that administers to the child's physical needs with a minimum of talking. While their needs are anticipated and responded to readily, there are few opportunities for children in this situation to experience repeated exposure to the same words or phrases. Additionally, the acceptability of nonverbal cues such as eye contact or gesture may vary. In some cultures, children learn quickly to avert their eyes when interacting with adults, a behavior that would appear deviant to the noncommunity observer.

Working Parents

In today's economy it is the rare family that does not have two working parents. This phenomenon has caused early intervention programs to redesign their formats to accommodate parents who must juggle economic necessity and family obligations. Parent/infant stimulation sessions must be scheduled creatively so that one or both parents, as well as the person designated as primary caregiver, can be present. In order to meet on a regular basis with the professional in a home-based or center-based program, the parent may need to arrange a flexible work schedule. As long as the parent is willing to spend quality time with the child before and after work, and the primary caregiver is committed to implementing aspects of the program, language learning is not compromised.

Nonparent Primary Caregiver

While the parent may have an intense desire to provide the stimulation required, it is unusual to find a babysitter, nanny, housekeeper, or day-care provider who has the same level of motivation. Since it is easy to credit the child's success or failure to the child-care provider, carrying out the program is a responsibility that many hourly employees are not anxious to assume. Thus, in addition to adjusting to the stresses and time commitment of having a hearing-impaired child, parents often have to radically change their child-care arrangements. For example, a day-care provider who speaks a language or dialect other than that which is acceptable in the community may need to be replaced by a person capable of providing appropriate language models during daily routines.

Parent Training Rationale

Approaches to Parent Education

A common approach is to educate parents about hearing loss, its impact on social and communicative performance, and potential educational options, as well as to deal with the emotional turmoil experienced at this early stage (Luterman, 1979), prior to making a final program decision. The result of this approach is that the parents defer decisions while they are acquiring the corpus of information necessary to choose programs, and their child remains unserved. It seems more appropriate to provide parents at the outset of a parent/infant training program with rudimentary information and general stimulation necessities that will be useful regardless of the educational program or communicative modality ultimately chosen. As the parents acquire new information they can modify the approach, modality, and program.

John Tracy Clinic's Home Correspondence course is an example of an approach to parent education that capitalizes on the parents' intrinsic desire to help their child. Although it attempts to adapt the program to the child's needs with a personal letter accompanying the appropriate "lesson" material, there is no on-site professional involved to assist in stimulating, eliciting, and reinforcing the concepts. The inventive parent can take the ideas and concepts suggested in the course and adapt them to a variety of situations that exist in the home. However, since a lesson is considered completed when the child has achieved a certain percent success rate, it is easy to imagine that a parent might do the lesson once or twice, consider it sufficient, and write for the next lesson in the sequence. With such an approach mastery of skills would be minimal.

The SKI HI program uses preset lessons to educate the parents about physical and functional aspects of hearing loss, the audiogram, professional personnel, amplification components and use, and language development. These lessons are "taught" by a parent advisor who makes regular visits to the home. Suggestions for stimulating language in children are made with accompanying material. However, the "scripts" that are written for the parent advisor do not account for differences in parenting style, child-rearing practices, educational level, interest, and motivation. The effectiveness of the child-stimulation activities are dependent on the skill level of the home visitor, who is not necessarily an aural rehabilitation specialist. Yet, the SKI HI program has filled a void in areas of the country where there are no trained professionals within commuting distance.

The message from both of these parent-infant programs is that parents are critical to the child's success regardless of the communication modality chosen. The programs give direction to parents at a time when they desperately need it. They provide an excellent program option, especially for families who live in rural areas where few direct services are available. The most effective method is to combine such generic parent education programs with a direct service approach, where a trained professional can help shape the child's behaviors and find the rate and complexity level of information that the particular parent can absorb.

Regardless of the approach used, there is a body of information applicable to all parents beginning the process:

amplification
    what it is and isn't
    necessity and use
parent/caregiver input
    quality and quantity
    effective use of the home environment
parents role over time

Home-based versus Center-based Programming

Parent/infant sessions can be home-based, or center-based in a school or rehabilitation facility. In home-based training, whatever is present in the home environment becomes the vehicle for language learning. Parents can learn to capitalize on the rich home environment by participating fully in the home sessions, which are designed to incorporate the speech/language objectives into daily routines. The home environment should not be used to carry out the same activities that would take place in a center. Without parent involvement, the home-based sessions would be merely displaced replicas of center-based sessions.

It is often too expensive for schools or rehabilitative agencies to conduct home-based programming. The amount of time required for the early intervention specialist to travel between homes limits the number of parents/children that can be seen in one day. Thus home-based programming is neither cost-efficient nor cost-effective, especially in rural areas.

A center-based program either requires the parents to transport the child to the center or provides transportation for the family with taxis, car service, or minibus. With the specialist located at one site, more families can avail themselves of the service. However, the numbers game does not tell the whole story. When a program takes place in the home, the attendance rate for each family improves since the specialist makes visits even during marginal weather and ill health. The effectiveness of center-based programming, on the other hand, depends on the commitment the parent brings to it. Therefore, although the overall number of scheduled visits per family is reduced for the home-based programs, the actual number of family specialist contacts may be similar for both sites.

The challenge in a center-based program is to creatively utilize the sterile clinic environment to duplicate the routines and activities that occur naturally in the home. During the parent/infant therapy sessions, the therapist can use dolls and doll furniture to represent the objects and people that are present in the home. The parent then becomes the vehicle for effectively transferring and implementing clinic goals within the home setting. To observe how much this has occurred, a home visit should be made at least once a year. The remainder of the time the therapist depends on the parent to report any difficulties he/she is having in accomplishing assigned tasks. Although clinic modifications that incorporate toys, dolls, and models are poor alternatives to carrying out therapy at the child's home, they are the only options within the space constraints of a clinic or school setting.

A more viable center-based option is to equip a room with the accouterments of a home. This creates the illusion of the therapist/parent/child interacting within a natural environment. By providing a realistic home setting, it is possible to increase the parent's proficiency in utilizing the natural environment for language learning.

That a program is center-based does not preclude intense parent involvement. Center-based programs should target words, phrases, and sentences that are required for function within the home, even without the real objects or daily routines at hand. Professionals should orchestrate situations in which such linguistic elements can be learned. Further, the parents must incorporate the techniques demonstrated during these clinic sessions into their daily routines.

Modifying Parent/Infant Interaction

Parent training is based on the following assumptions: (1) language learning takes place in the home, where the daily routines are the topics, and the mundane, repetitive phrases are the first learned; (2) the time that the parent and child spend with the professional is only sufficient to guide and direct skills, not to establish and stabilize them; (3) caregivers in the home environment play the major role in implementing the goals and objectives; and (4) it is possible to train parents/caregivers to provide effective and efficient language stimulation in the home environment.

Given the above framework, the next step is to determine the most effective approach to help parents enhance and/or modify their own communicative behaviors so that maximum benefit is obtained. It is important to individualize parent training according to parenting style, behavioral management approach, availability of multiple caregivers, and time commitment.

Parent Education Strategies

All the approaches shown in Table 5.4 assume that the parent needs to be informed and educated. Approaches (a) and (b) are an integral part of any program, yet they are ineffective when used as the only means of training parents. It is difficult for parents to take the general information presented in these curricula or philosophical treatises and apply it to their own situation. Yet the material does provide inspiration and motivation during a time when parents may be discouraged about slow progress.

Approaches (c) to (g) represent varying degrees of parent involvement during the training sessions. Many professionals organize sessions into two components: time spent with the child attempting to establish skills, and time spent explaining to

Table 5.4 List of the typical approaches to parent training utilized in existing parent/infant programs.

a.	reading
b.	lecture
c.	describe what happened and what should be done
d.	observe outside of the therapy room
e.	observe inside therapy room
f.	participate in session
g.	provide direct instruction during the session

the parents what happened during the session and how to carry it over to the home (c,d,e). Since the parents may not have any opportunity to observe the activities while in session, extensive explanation may be necessary. Others may have observed the session from outside or inside the therapy room but at a distance from the activity. Observational approaches assume that the parents will be able to emulate the techniques employed by the professional

when they interact with their child in the home environment. These observational approaches thus prepare the parents to provide structured "lessons" at home.

Optimally, the parents will absorb the techniques that have been demonstrated into their own unique interaction style. This result is best achieved by letting them participate actively in each session (f,g). The highest level of involvement occurs when parents receive instruction while codirecting the therapy activity—instead of trying to replicate the professional's teaching style, they are helped to optimize their own.

Whenever parents are involved, it is important to fine-tune their observation skills since they become the primary reporter of the child's language use at home. Knowing what happens day to day becomes the yardstick against which other test results and observations are measured. Time educating the parent is therefore well spent. They need to be aware of the complexity of the language as well as the acoustic characteristics of the stimulus, as illustrated in Table 5.5.

Although parents express their intention to change their auditory/linguistic expectations, it is difficult to change long-standing habits. Most parents are unaware of the extent to which they have accommodated the communicative needs of their infants. Parents should not only be verbally instructed about changes needed in their interaction style, but also practice those changes with the child as the professional

Table 5.5 Analysis of the child's response requires knowledge of the acoustics of the stimulus, the contextual support present, and the child's attention to stimuli.

1. CHARACTERISTICS OF THE STIMULUS
    Acoustic Parameters
        intonation, rhythm, duration, phonemes
    Linguistic Complexity
        vocabulary, syntax, familiarity

2. CONTEXTUAL SUPPORT
    Situational
        departure, greeting, referent present
    Linguistic
        predictability from sentence structure and meaning

3. ATTENTION TO STIMULI
    Level of involvement, distractibility

4. REPEATABILITY

observes. Videotaped parent/child interactions can become a learning experience if the professional helps parents observe their interactions.

SPEECH/LANGUAGE ACQUISITION

As long as the speech signal is audible to the child, a normal progression of spoken language development is possible. The degree of audibility is often the key to the learning process. At one end of the continuum are the children with mild to moderate hearing losses who are able to develop spoken language from exposure to speech from peers and adults. For them, remedial activities include "fine-tuning" their language skills, broadening the knowledge that is already present, and hastening the language learning process.

The children with more severe hearing losses need more than exposure to linguistic forms and vocabulary to deduce the rules of language. For these children, adults must purposefully organize their input to facilitate the sequential, integrated development of auditory, speech, and language skills. The success of this endeavor depends on the knowledge and expectations of the rehabilitation provider and parents, the child's innate intelligence, and the age that full-time amplification began.

A key ingredient in this process is a caregiver who can capitalize on every activity as a potential vehicle for learning language. The ability to use hearing to deduce meaning occurs within the context of conversation associated with daily activities rather than "through auditory training divorced from meaningful contexts" (Patersen, 1986). Daily routines such as eating, playing, diapering, and bathing, in addition to their usual value to the child, take on a new dimension when viewed as a language learning tool. Since these activities occur frequently in the child's life, they naturally provide the repetition required for learning to happen (Mischook and Cole, 1986). For example, each meal may be used to teach *vocabulary* (cheese, milk, cereal), introduce *action verbs* (cutting, stirring, throwing), obligate use of *grammar* (plural /s/ in "two bites"; possessive /z/ in "Mommy's"), and present *social phrases* ("Pay attention"; "Just one more".)

Auditory skill development does not develop in isolation in normally hearing children. Therapeutic strategies that train isolated skills in hearing-impaired children are thus counterintuitive. The most rapid development of spoken language occurs when audition/speech/language are thought of as a single unit with interdependent objectives and goals. For example, when a normally hearing infant begins to produce a particular phoneme in his/her babbling, he/she is simultaneously auditorally distinguishing among that phoneme and others that vary in the numbers of shared distinctive features. As the phoneme is repeated frequently in the child's babbling, it takes on meaning when it occurs many times in association with the same person, object, or event. Thus speech, language, and listening have developed simultaneously in a meaningful context.

Table 5.6 displays the interrelationship of auditory, speech, and language goals during an age-appropriate activity or routine. Using this integrated approach, it is possible to sample the child's auditory perception of suprasegmental and segmental aspects of speech, provide gradually more difficult acoustic contrasts to identify, expose the child to unfamiliar vocabulary or linguistic forms as well as situations that obligate their use, and train auditory monitoring of speech skills. In this example the situational context could be the daily routines of sleeping and eating using a baby doll and a stuffed cat.

Incidental verbal learning is negligible for profoundly hearing-impaired children in the early stages of language learning. In order for learning to occur, the child needs many meaningful opportunities to use or act on what is being said. For example, using a stimulating context of dressing the child, /sh/ can be heard or used multiple times in the words *shirt, shorts, wash, shoes, shoelaces, shine your shoes, undershirt, washcloth.* Most important is that the target repeatedly occurs in situational contexts relevant to the child's life experience, such as those that occur daily during home routines.

EDUCATION

Much of early learning derives from watching, analyzing, and interacting with other children. The most socially integrated children are those that have had many opportunities to interact with peers. A formal program does not have to be established to provide a social environment—parents can turn their own social outings into learning experiences. This does not mean that they have to intervene between children to encourage language learning; rather, such informal gatherings expose children to social interactions and lay the groundwork for coping with future social demands.

Table 5.6   Speech, language, and auditory development are intertwined-not worked on as separate entities.

Language	Speech	Audition
Adult presents:	Adult presents: baby	Adult presents:
Child uses:	Child repeats: baby	Child act or repeats:
baby	if /ee/ in baby is poor,	where baby (intonation)
(let's) play with baby	the adult stresses /ee/	baby vs. cat (syllable #)
where's (the) baby	the next time baby is	sound association for cat
(the) baby's crying	called ("babEE") -	and baby (meow vs. wah)
(the) baby fell down	child repeats using	baby vs. mommy (on vowel)
	corrected sound	

In the past it would have been unnecessary to discuss "out-of-the-home" programs for hearing-impaired infants since fewer homes had two working parents. In today's economic climate, however, more children are spending part of their day in group child care or with a nonparent caregiver. When there is a choice, however, many parents prefer to keep their hearing-impaired infants in the more protected home environment rather than expose them to the demands of a play group under the direction of a nonparent adult.

INFANT AUDITORY MANAGEMENT

For the infant with normal hearing, auditory perceptual development begins the first day of life, if not earlier. Every day that hearing loss is unidentified and amplification delayed, the hearing-impaired child loses valuable speech/language acquisition time.

Auditory perceptual skills range from simple detection (presence versus absence of sound), to identification (label the sound), to discrimination (perceive the difference between sounds). Without these basic auditory skills, a child cannot cope with the complex auditory stimuli necessary for perceiving speech.

Early perceptual development occurs according to the following hierarchy:

1. Assimilation tendencies and contrast effects increase with increasing age.
2. Younger children fail to relate a stimulus to the spatial framework in which it appears.
3. Younger children require greater redundancy in a pattern to perceive it correctly. Incomplete or complex patterns are difficult for younger children.
4. Dependency on multiple cues in constancies decreases with increasing age.

Parents/caregivers need to be informed about the stages of auditory development that precede comprehension of words or the production of the first word. Table 5.7 may be helpful in guiding nonprofessionals through the early, difficult stages of communication development.

Selection and Fitting of Amplification

The first step in auditory management is providing amplification. The older the child, the easier it is to decide the best type of hearing aid and its appropriate electroacoustic characteristics. However, the process cannot be delayed until it becomes "easy." Selection and fitting of amplification is an ongoing process for infants and toddlers. Although the clinical audiologist is responsible for making the final decisions, he/she cannot conduct an appropriate hearing aid evaluation without the informed coop-

Table 5.7   Summary of auditory development in the normally hearing infant.

Skill	Age	Behavioral Manifestations
Horizontal localization	0-3 months	Gross movement toward source
	4-6 months	Direct movement on lateral plane
	7 months +	Direct movement in all planes
Minimal Audible Angle	6-18 months	Decreases from 15 to 4 degrees
Detection of duration differences	<6 months	Difference must be at least 20 msec for detection
Pitch perception	<6 months	Differences must be large for detection
Speech perception	1 month	VOT discriminations (pa vs. ba) can be made
	2 months	Can differentiate phonemes with falling fundamental frequency versus a rising one
	9 months	Very attentive to mother's natural voice
	9-18 months	Prefer low redundancy highly novel speech segments

eration of other professionals working with the child and parents/caregivers. The purpose of conducting evaluations in the controlled environment of the clinic is to assess amplification function and benefit. However, aided performance in the optimal conditions (quiet, close to the sound source, controlled signals) of the sound-proof booth does not necessarily predict equally good performance in everyday listening situations. Further, since infants and toddlers cannot report subjective responses, the standardized techniques that yield such practical information with older children and adults are inappropriate for the 0–3-year-old. Only through the cooperative efforts of family and professionals can the adequacy of the speech signal reaching the child's ear and the possibility of over- or underamplification be determined.

Hearing Aid Evaluation (HAE)

Although a valid hearing aid evaluation depends on the availability of audiological data, infants and toddlers can be appropriately fit with only basic information (Maxon, 1987; Maxon and Smaldino, 1991). A child can be fit initially using sound field frequency-specific minimal awareness levels (MAL), including a target audiogram (250, 1000, 4000 Hz) and Speech Awareness Threshold/Music Threshold. At four months and older, infants can localize a sound source at low sensation levels. When there is a minimal difference in between-ear sensitivity the observable responses allow for a binaural fitting. With as little as 500 Hz and 2000 Hz MAL a flexible hearing aid can be provided (Beauchaine, Barlow, and Stelmachowicz, 1990).

The child with a severe to profound hearing loss may not be able to give unaided responses because the audiometer does not produce signals that are loud enough to be salient. Lack of unaided responses should not be interpreted as the child's inability to benefit from traditional amplification. Instead, binaural, high-gain hearing aids or a personal FM system should be provided during a carefully designed trial to allow the child auditory experiences.

Once hearing aids (or an FM system) have been selected, the fitting process must take place. The clinical assessment component should be conducted only after the child has used amplification on a full-time basis for at least two weeks. During that time the child will become accustomed to receiving sound, and test results will likely be a more accurate reflection of the benefits or weaknesses of the fitting.

Audiologically, appropriate gain, output, and frequency response are the basic considerations of amplification fitting (see Chapter 2). Refinement of those characteristics may not be easily achieved with the infant or toddler, but it is possible to make sound audible across the speech frequency range without making it intolerably loud (Beauchaine, Barlow, and Stelmachowicz, 1990).

Since a primary goal of amplification is to ensure that the child has access to suprathreshold sounds, especially speech, unaided and aided performance can provide invaluable information about functional benefits. A simple comparison of aided and unaided responses to their names, music, or mothers' voices can be used for younger children or those with lower language levels. Older toddlers may follow simple commands. An estimate of the range of audible speech sounds can be made using Ling's (1976) 5-sound (a, i, u, s, sh) test or the Early Speech Perception (ESP) test (Moog and Geers, 1988).

Some audiologists are more comfortable with what they consider objective techniques. Use of real ear measures and formula-based techniques have potential for determining hearing aid electroacoustic characteristics for infants and toddlers. A formula-based approach enables the audiologist to predict the sound that will actually be delivered to the child's ear. Desired Sensation Level method accounts for the higher sound pressure levels and resonance peaks of the external ear canals of children under the age of two years (Seewald and Ross, 1988). A simple formula can be used to select an appropriate output level (SSPL-90). For infants and toddlers, 100dB +1/4 of the MALs (dB HL) at 1000, 2000, 4000 Hz - 10dB gives the average output at which hearing aids should be set. This formula takes into account the differences in ear canal volume for young children as compared to adults (Bebout, (1989). In any formula-based approach, very specific numbers can be obtained, but the child's abilities cannot be determined. The estimates are helpful, but should not be the basis on which any final, long-term decisions are made.

A monitored trial like that prescribed in the SKI HI home program (Clark and Watkins, 1978) or the less formal loaner period prescribed by Maxon (1981) is crucial for establishing appropriateness of amplification. In this way, gain, frequency response, and output setting refinement decisions are made with the child as the base, rather than from a predictive model.

The child's behavior using amplification in the everyday environment is the key to determining benefit. Table 5.8 displays how SSPL-90 settings affect a child's reaction to loud and moderate-level sounds (environmental, others' speech, own speech). It is particularly important to ensure that the child is not overamplified, but underamplification is also a problem that should not be overlooked. To assess the correctness of gain settings, responses (alerting, localization, distance differences) to moderate- and low-level sounds are monitored and any necessary changes made.

With adults, frequency response is viewed as crucial for a good hearing aid fit. Since it is more difficult to judge appropriateness of amplification across frequencies with infants and toddlers, its importance may be ignored. Merely looking for a child's reaction to his/her name will not indicate which frequency components the child hears. Availability of the speech signal should encompass the access to the various acoustic cues of speech as well as audibility. For example, low-frequency energy is required for the development of the suprasegmental features of speech, but lack of high-frequency cues impacts on speech perception, production, and syntactic development. Parents/caregivers must therefore learn to observe and differentiate among a child's responses to environmental sounds, broad spectrum speech, and frequency-specific speech sounds. Poor responses to particular frequency bands may indicate that the electroacoustic characteristic settings of the hearing aids should be tested.

FM systems are used most often in classrooms, but there has been an increase in their use as primary amplification for young children. Not every infant and toddler is a candidate for an FM fitting. The purpose of using the FM system is to provide a good speech signal in less-than-optimal signal-to-noise ratios. This becomes particularly critical for the child with profound hearing loss in learning language when the various semantic, syntactic, and phonological rules are being deduced. The child with hearing loss is always at a disadvantage when accessing speech. However, profound hearing loss makes it virtually impossible for the child to have any access without a quiet background and very close proximity to the sound source.

The use of an FM system as personal amplification allows the parent/caregiver to carry out typical everyday tasks and provide the child with a good, clear signal. For example, in a breakfast preparation routine containing two school-age children discussing their activities and an infant seated across the room in a high chair, the parent can easily talk to the child with hearing loss, describing and reporting on the food preparation and providing good language input during the regular course of the family setting. If the parent uses an FM system, the same input can be provided without requiring that the other children remain quiet.

Table 5.8 Responses to auditory stimuli that provide cues to appropriateness of amplification fitting.

Behavior	Indication
BLINKING/FLINCHING	
to moderately loud sounds	Output (SSPL-90) too high
	Gain too high
	Unwanted output peaks
to lower frequency sounds	Overamplification in lows
TURNING	
to common environmental sounds	
to conversational speech	Appropriate gain
to name being called	
ALERTING	
to higher-frequency sounds	Good high-frequency response
to lower-frequency sounds	Good low-frequency response
to general speech	Good gain and frequency response
NO RESPONSE	
to common environmental sounds	
to conversational speech	Gain too low
to name being called	
SPEECH SOUNDS	
restricted to voiced/vowel sounds	Inappropriate frequency response
monotonous	
include voiceless sounds	Appropriate frequency response
variable (age appropriate)	

When a child is a candidate for an FM system as primary amplification, it is critical to ensure that the child can benefit from it and that the family can accommodate it. Through a careful program like that shown in Table 5.1, the professionals and family can establish the best way to use the FM system. Since FM use with an infant/toddler is not limited to one setting, it is necessary to assess the benefits in various settings, such as at home, out shopping, at the home of friends and relatives, and on the playground.

Troubleshooting Amplification

An important component of early auditory management is training parents/caregivers to monitor their child's amplification. The professional (audiologist, speech-language pathologist, teacher of the hearing impaired) who educates them provides the necessary equipment (battery tester, stethoscope, etc.) and method for charting results, and demonstrates how to make simple repairs. (A complete troubleshooting protocol for various types of amplification is provided in the Appendix.) Monitoring amplification function should also include continued observation to identify changes in the child's auditory, vocal, and general behavior that indicate amplification malfunction and/or changes in the previously documented benefit.

Monitoring and Refining the Fitting

The process of learning spoken language begins when the child receives audible speech, i.e., at suprathreshold levels. In some cases this may be when the amplification is first fit, and for others it may take several revisions before the appropriate settings are determined. To avoid unnecessary delays in amplification, the fitting should be monitored closely for the first few months until the parent and audiologist are convinced that the child is responding at optimal levels across speech frequencies given the degree and configuration of the hearing loss.

Too often, audiologists take a conservative approach to fitting to avoid overamplification, setting up the parents for low auditory expectations. Then, if no auditory response is forthcoming the parents may fear that the hearing loss has gotten worse, or is unaidable and experience grief for a second time. They rightfully want to know that there are benefits to wearing this highly visible device—that he/she can hear. The parents need to observe concrete realistic behaviors during this initial adjustment period. If the parents of a profoundly deaf child are expecting to see consistent, repeatable responses to speech during the first weeks, they will likely become frustrated and perhaps reduce the intensity of their efforts. If, on the other hand, they are advised to look for a listening attitude, a decrease/increase in vocalization, or quieting or cessation of movement when a loud, low-frequency sound appears, it is much more likely that they will observe this behavior and be rewarded for their efforts.

Immediate full-time usage is critical. Suggesting that the child gradually increase his/her amplification usage over a period of several weeks or months will only lead to problems. Only when the parents are convinced that the child needs the amplification and are willing to provide it will full-time use become routine. If the parents are still feeling sorry for the child, it will be very difficult for them to insist that the child wear the amplification. The older the child at the time amplification is introduced, the more assertive the parents need to be. Acceptance of amplification occurs most rapidly between zero and fourteen months, children between fifteen months and three years may put up a struggle. Therefore, parents must be thoroughly prepared for a battle, realizing that any ambivalence about amplification on their part will be obvious to the discerning preschooler. They should be ready with ways of distracting their child from a typical, single-minded course of action—pulling out the earmolds. Although difficult, a two-day initial struggle in which full-time usage is demanded eliminates a month-long battle, the results for part-time usage.

HINTS:
- keep both hands occupied with food, toys
- have an exciting activity available
- make sure the ear-level aid is not flopping off the ear
- make sure that body aid or FM cords are out of sight and reach
- if hearing aid is taken out, replace it immediately
- only an adult removes the hearing aid for naps, bath, etc.
- the adult is in charge

An immediate concern for parents is how best to inform family members about the hearing loss and hearing aids. Practicing explanations can help parents feel more comfortable at a time when they are not completely informed themselves and are vulnerable to criticism and other people's opinions. A particularly traumatic time occurs when they take their first excursion outside of the home with their child. They are unsure of the best response when people express sympathy and give unsolicited advice. They should be aware that a simple description of the equipment and a statement about their satisfaction in finding a management program that meets their needs should silence the critics and the curious. Later, as they become more expert in the effects of hearing loss, they will be more competent in fielding questions and educating the community.

Awareness of Listening Environment

To assume hearing problems are remedied by amplification gives parents of newly identified infants a false sense of security. They must learn that listening conditions common to the daily environment compromise the utility of amplification systems. Although the home environment typically has sound-absorbing surfaces and materials that reduce reverberation and noise, there remain many opportunities for the speech input from caregivers to be compromised by internal and external noise. The same daily routines that provide the most fodder for discussion have the potential to produce the greatest amount of noise. For example, food preparation, dishwashing, and laundry activities all involve noisy appliances. In order to effectively use these routines, parents need to be aware of the noise potential and to time their verbal inputs to those moments preceding and following the use of the equipment. When the television is on or other siblings are making noise, the infant is less likely to hear the speech of the caregiver and to respond appropriately.

Noise

Internal	External
appliances	car
large group	street noise
media	heavy equipment
siblings	animals
friends	playground

To further complicate the situation, once infants are ambulatory, the distances between them and their caregivers increase, decreasing the intensity of the speech that reaches them. Therefore, although increased mobility gives the parent and child infinitely more to talk about and react to, it also interferes with the audibility of the signal. Toddlers are often fifteen to twenty feet from the talker whether they are in the same room, in a different room, or on another floor. Distance further interferes with speech reception when the listening environment is noisy.

Boothroyd (1988) developed an equation which capsulizes the auditory learning situation (see Table 5.9). Auditory capacity is composed of optimal, functional amplification and the listening condition. Exploiting this auditory potential becomes the caregivers' job. They must find or develop many opportunities for learning within daily routines if they expect the child to fully utilize the sound. The less auditory capacity available, the more frequent the learning opportunities need to be. Conversely, the child with a lesser degree of hearing loss requires fewer examples of the sound in a context before optimal auditory performance results.

Helping parents be effective in their effort to develop optimal auditory performance is a two-step process. First, they need to set realistic expectations depending on their child's age, degree of hearing loss, and time since wearing amplification full-time. The second step is to provide them with the means to facilitate auditory development to meet their level of expectation. The more severe the hearing impairment, the more necessary it is to train the skill rather than to wait for it to emerge. Thus,

Table 5.9 A description of the components involved in optimizing auditory performance.

Auditory Capacity	×	Learning Opportunities	= Auditory Performance
limited	×	excellent	= good to excellent
excellent	×	excellent	= excellent
limited	×	limited	= poor
excellent	×	limited	= fair

in addition to providing a rich auditory environment under optimal listening conditions, parents must help the child learn to depend on the cues to which he/she has access.

Another aspect of auditory learning that falls to parents is establishing the child as responsible for his/her own hearing. This requires that the infant learn to push in the earmolds when they become unseated and to ask an adult's assistance to replace an ear-level hearing aid or a button receiver when it falls out. Also, the child should be responsible for indicating when the amplification is malfunctioning, or has no sound or a barely audible signal.

SUMMARY

A hearing loss identified in an infant has enormous communicative and social ramifications for the child and family. For the child, it means that he/she will require years of communication training in order to develop intelligible speech and good language. For the parents, it means years of working intensively with their child, attempting to linguistically enhance every activity, routine, or event in which the child is involved.

References

Beauchaine, K., Barlow, N. & Stelmachowicz, P. (1990). Special considerations in amplification for young children. *ASHA* 32, 44-46.

Bebout, J. (1989). Pediatric hearing aid fitting: A practical overview. *Hearing Journal* 42, 8, 13-20.

Boothroyd, A. (1988). *Hearing Impairment in Young Children.* Washington, DC: A. G. Bell Association.

Clark, T.C. & Watkins, S. (1978). *Programming for Hearing-Impaired Infants Through Amplification and Intervention,* The SKI HI Model.

Cole, E. and St. Clair-Stokes, J. (1984). Caregiver-child interactive behaviors: A videotape analysis procedure. *Volta Review*, 86, 4, 200-216.

Ling, D. (1976). *Speech and the Hearing-Impaired Child: Theory and Practice.* Washington, DC: A.G. Bell Association.

Luterman, D. (1979). *Counseling Parents of Hearing-Impaired Children.* Boston, MA: Little, Brown and Company.

Maxon, A.B. (1981). Speech acoustics: A model for managing the hearing-impaired child. Paper presented at ASHA, Toronto, Canada.

Maxon, A.B. (1987). Pediatric amplification. In F.N. Martin (Ed.) *Hearing Disorders in Children* (pp. 361-395). Austin, TX: Pro-Ed.

Maxon, A.B. & Smaldino, J. (1991). Hearing aid management for children. *Seminars in Hearing.*

Mischook, M. & Cole, E. (1986). Auditory learning and teaching of hearing-impaired infants. In E. Cole & H. Gregory (Eds.) *Auditory Learning, Volta Review* 88, 5.

Moog, J. & Geers, A. (1988). *Early Speech Perception Test.* St. Louis, MO: Central Institute for the Deaf.

Patersen, M. (1986). Maximizing the use of residual hearing with school-aged hearing-impaired students - A perspective. In E. Cole & H. Gregory (Eds.) *Auditory Learning, Volta Review* 88, 93-108.

Seewald, R.C. & Ross, M. (1988). Amplification for the young hearing-impaired child. In M. Pollack (Ed.) *Amplification for the Hearing Impaired*. New York NY: Grunt and Stratton, (pp. 213-267).

6

Programming: Preschoolers (3–5 years)

INTRODUCTION

The need to emphasize the child's social or academic communication changes with his/her chronological age. In the preschool years the social aspects of communication predominate, since the goal of early childhood education is to prepare the child for social interactions within a group. Once the hearing-impaired student becomes school age, there is a more equal balance between social requirements and academic necessities.

PROGRAMMING CONSIDERATIONS

As the child approaches age three, decisions must be made regarding the preschool educational placement. Two distinct options exist: a self-contained class or a mainstream preschool; a third option comprises a combination of the two.

With a mainstream option, the parents will have selected a stimulating early childhood program that conforms to certain acoustic and linguistic criteria and allows for school visits, use of equipment, and curriculum preview. Such a placement assumes that the child has the social and communicative skills to benefit from a highly verbal environment. The child's social group is normally hearing same-age peers with age-appropriate speech and language skills. The parents' responsibility is increased as they prepare their child for the language of social interactions and academics (see Table 6.1).

The second alternative is to locate a preschool program specially designed for hearing-impaired children. Selection may be based on availability, communicative modality, family involvement, curriculum, and amplification use. The trained teacher who understands the communicative needs of this population becomes the primary source of language input, with parents reinforcing class concepts. The child's social group is hearing-impaired similarly aged peers with speech and language deficits (see Table 6.1).

Table 6.1   Typical characteristics of preschool classes options for hearing-impaired students.

	Mainstream Class	*Self-Contained Class*
number of students	12-20	8 maximum
teacher/student ratio	8:1	4:1
acoustic treatment	potentially none	typically present
teacher modifications	potentially none	typically present
language comparison	normally hearing	hearing-impaired
speech comparison	normally hearing	hearing-impaired
social comparison	normally hearing	hearing-impaired
academic skills	normally hearing	normally hearing
quality of peer/peer communication	good	poor
parent involvement	good	limited

The third alternative applies when the child is enrolled simultaneously in a specialized preschool and a mainstream early childhood program. In such a dual-focus program the child is exposed to the demands of a mainstream placement while benefiting from the structure of a language-based class. With such an arrangement the parents need to preview the concepts of the mainstream class as well as work on the remedial activities of the self-contained classroom.

MAINSTREAM PRESCHOOL PLACEMENT

Consideration of a mainstream early childhood program as a placement for a hearing-impaired preschooler is appropriate when the child has a sufficient foundation to benefit from exposure to normal social, academic, and communicative behavior. Specifically, the child must be motivated to emulate the behaviors exhibited by his/her classmates as they interact with each other and the teacher.

Characteristics of Students

Auditory Skills

To access the verbal information of the class, the preschooler must know when someone is talking to him/her. This basic level of detection should be automatic by the time the child enters the class. With more advanced word recognition skills, the student can hear the actual words the other students use as they socially interact during early childhood activities. When no response to sound is evident, the teacher and peers will have to make major modifications to obtain the hearing-impaired child's attention and verbal interaction.

Speech Skills

It is expected that the hearing-impaired three-year-old entering an organized preschool for the first time will have delays in speech and language. The words/phrases that the child says should be recognizable to the teacher and peers within the situational context. This does not mean that they must be perfectly articulated or recognizable without the framework of the interaction or activity.

Language Skills

To fully benefit from the language-rich environment, hearing-impaired preschoolers should optimally be generating two-word combinations. While this leaves them at a disadvantage compared to their peers who are at the full-sentence stage, it provides a foundation on which to build sentence structure and insert new vocabulary. The preschooler who is only at the single-word level still has to deduce the effectiveness of word combinations to express ideas. Although exposure to the sentence-length utterance of the other students may facilitate the emergence of these combinations, it also may prove to be so complex that the child cannot extract the pertinent elements required to build the simple combinations.

Social Skills

The preschooler entering a mainstream early childhood program must be able to function as part of a group and to learn from a nonparent adult. The most important social prerequisites are the desire to be with peers and motivation to participate and interact.

Parent Involvement

Since the student is in school for only a few hours a week (two days = six hours/week), parents, with the guidance of trained professionals, remain the primary source of input. If this option is chosen, the parent has a major responsibility to continue to provide intensive speech/language/listening training within the home environment.

Service Provision

For the mainstream option all the special services are conducted outside of the education setting unless some special arrangement is made through the private early childhood center. Occasionally a state-supported nursery school will have speech/language services on site or be willing to contract for them. As long as in-service training is provided these programs can be effective.

Auditory Support

Auditory management for the mainstreamed preschool child begins with analyzing the listening environment for potentially disruptive noise sources. This task is best accomplished by unobtrusively observing the class in session, with the full complement of children present. Obtaining a verbal description of the classroom activities is insufficient since it does not indicate how the activity is used. Table 6.2 categorizes preschool activities according to typical use pattern. The need for observation can be appreciated by seeing that in a particular early childhood program, "snack" is considered a quiet, noninteractive activity, putting it in the Group/Quiet category.

When activities generate noise either through manipulation of equipment or through verbal interaction, a carpet or carpet remnant can be placed in the noisy area to help with sound absorption. Some parents have been willing to provide carpeting to a school in order that their child better hear his/her teacher and classmates. An alternative is to solicit area carpet stores to donate remnants to the school. They can use such donations as a tax write-off. Carpeting is the single most effective classroom

Table 6.2   Analysis of the noise generated in individual and group activities typical of preschool programs.

Environmental Analysis

	Individual	*Group*
Quiet	reading arts+crafts puzzles	circle cooking story show and tell
Noise	blocks carpentry	housekeeping corner trucks snack songs musical instruments

modification available—it can reduce ambient noise levels by as much as 20dB. When a school does not have carpeting, there are ways to find funding for it.

Through classroom observation it will also become clear when distance interacts with noise to negatively affect speech reception. Teachers typically organize the structured group times in a physical arrangement that facilitates maximum visibility and audibility. If a circle is maintained for attendance, calendar, and greeting time, the hearing-impaired child can be placed at the equivalent of 3 o'clock or 9 o'clock, with the teacher sitting at 12 o'clock. In this way the child is close enough to hear the teacher and to see his/her face, as well as any other visual display that is used. If loosely defined rows are used instead, the child should sit in front of the teacher or at a forty-five-degree angle to him/her. The slightly off-center placement allows the child a better view of his/her classmates when they are responding.

Attention to such modifications provides hearing-impaired students an opportunity to use their best listening skills and participate fully in preschool life. Without them, they receive a very poor auditory signal and must resort primarily to visual reception of speech.

Visual Support

The teacher may need to make minor modifications in teaching style to further enhance the reception of speech. In preschool programs teachers use visual displays to provide associations for the words being said. They hold up objects, demonstrate a movement, or show a picture that supplements the songs, stories, or other words. Using visual displays particularly helps the hearing-impaired student who enters the preschool exhibiting a linguistic deficit. Any supplementary information clearly enhances the child's ability to ascertain meaning. However, although visual demonstration helps, it also produces a situation in which speech reception is compromised. By shifting the child's visual attention to the picture or object, his/her visual focus is transferred away from the teacher's face, where speechreading cues are present. He/she must then rely entirely on the quality of auditory input for the reception of information. If the room is noisy or the teacher is seated at a less-than-optimal distance, a partial or at best pieced-together message is received.

The teacher can vary his/her rhythm to accommodate the child's need to receive full auditory/visual speech input as well as to look at the visual display, and so reduce the potential for this communication breakdown. For example, the pattern can be LOOK (at visual display)-LOOK/LISTEN (at face for explanation)-LOOK (at visual display for further confirmation). An alternative approach is LOOK/LISTEN (at the face for the explanation) and LOOK (at the visual display). The teacher can control the visual focus of the class by directing his/her own eye gaze at the visual display when appropriate, and at the class when the students should be looking at him/her.

Media

Preschool programs frequently use media such as records and/or audiotapes to supplement the music, movement, or story aspects of the curriculum. Usually the children listen to the material and perform some action related to it. The hearing-impaired student is obviously at a disadvantage when performance is dependent on "hearing" the instructions from an audio-only presentation. To circumvent this difficulty the teacher can send a list of the key words home for the parent to review prior to the lesson that relies on the media presentation in the classroom. This approach prepares the student to participate in the activity with the other students. If the student uses an FM system, the presentation can be enhanced by placing the FM microphone/transmitter on or near the loudspeaker of the record player or tape recorder. If the child does not have an FM unit, he/she can take a position close to the loudspeaker. The signal can be further reinforced when the teacher sings the words along with the record so that the child can hear and see the words at the same time.

Parent Involvement

Parents play several important roles when their children are enrolled in mainstream preschool placements. They act as liaison between the classroom teacher and the rehabilitation provider since these professionals are rarely at the same site. In this role they, with the teacher's assistance, identify the vocabulary and concepts to be used during upcoming activities and transmit this information to the aural rehabilitation provider, who will incorporate it into individual sessions. Parents also must inquire about the child's performance relative to his/her peers in specified activities, such as story time, circle, attendance, housekeeping corner, etc. With this information the parents and professionals can evaluate progress. Before the school experience begins, the teacher, aural rehabilitation specialist, and parent need to devise a system for communicating about the material to be previewed and reviewed at home. Often classroom teachers are reluctant to give the information requested ahead of time, rationalizing that none of the children totally understand the material at the time of presentation. The class is expected to gain familiarity with the vocabulary/concepts so that the next time they hear the words they will recognize them and associate them with the appropriate topic. Although this approach to learning is feasible for normally hearing children, the hearing-impaired preschooler enters the class without the linguistic foundation to pair with words and concepts. In order to improve linguistic competency the hearing-impaired child must master, not just be exposed to, the rich variety of words/concepts that occur in this setting. Since the necessary repetition cannot take place in the regular classroom, it must be reinforced by the aural rehabilitation specialist and parents.

Since the time the child actually spends in the classroom is minimal compared to home stimulation time, the parents' involvement in the child's day-to-day exposure and mastery of language continues to be primary. One of the benefits of placing children in a mainstream preschool is their exposure to a more varied vocabulary than is used at home. Much of the classroom curriculum is presented during the child's exploration of the materials or during repetitive formats such as circle time. Since preschool children do not read, there is little opportunity to depend on worksheets to support the concepts. Without input from the teachers, parents may thus find it difficult to identify and reinforce the actual units, vocabulary, and concepts being covered.

Under the guidance of an aural rehabilitation specialist, most parents can find creative ways of introducing the school concepts into daily routines and of exposing the child to general language appropriate to his/her age. Although the activities that occur in the home and school are different (see Table 6.3), the vocabulary and concepts overlap (see Table 6.4).

Teacher In-service

There are a variety of formats through which advice or suggestions can be transmitted to the teacher. General information can be given through reading material or a one-to-one encounter with the professional. In any format it is important to stress what the child has to offer the class and the kind of preparation that the child is getting for the classroom experience. The teacher may initially be skeptical about the efficacy of such a placement since it is unlikely that the preschooler will have language skills commensurate with his/her same-aged peers. Yet if the teacher recognizes the ultimate goal of this first school placement—to prepare the child to handle the communicative demands of the normally hearing world—he/she will join the

Table 6.3   Listing of home and school activities to be used for language stimulation.

Home Activities	*School Activities*
1. dressing for the day	1. attendance
2. dressing for outside	2. free play
3. doing laundry	3. housekeeping corner
4. loading the dishwasher	4. block building
5. rinsing/washing the dishes	5. snack time
6. changing diapers	6. story
7. setting the table	7. circle
8. preparing meals	8. songs
9. picking up toys	9. playground/recess
10. driving the car	10. arts and crafts
11. eating at a restaurant	11. greeting/departure
12. eating meals at home	12. free play
13. blowing nose	13. bathroom
14. preparing for bedtime	
15. preparing for bath	
16. wrapping presents	

Table 6.4   Examples of home and school dialogues based on common vocabulary/concepts.

Vocabulary/Concept:	CUP
Home:	Put the cup in the dishwasher.
	Get the cup for the juice.
	Oh no, you dropped your cup.
	Which cup do you want?
School:	Who wants a cup?
	Whose cup is this?
	Who didn't throw their cup away?
	Whose turn is it to pass out the cups?
	Who didn't get a cup?
Vocabulary/Concept:	CUTTING
Home:	Can you find something to cut with in the box?
	What can we use to cut the meat?
	That knife is too dull. Find a sharp one.
	You cut yourself.
	We need scissors to cut the wrapping paper.
School:	Did everyone get scissors to cut with?
	You need to cut on the dotted line.
Vocabulary/Concept:	CALENDAR (days/months/seasons)
Home:	Today is_____. Do we go to school?
	Tomorrow is _____. You have to go to bed early.
	In one more month, it will be your birthday.
	You can't wear that jacket. It's for winter.
	Let's check the calendar to see how many more days or months before we see Grandma.
School:	It's your turn to do Calendar.
	Who knows what day it is?
	In winter you wear_____; in spring you wear_____.
	Who has a birthday in January?

effort. Many teachers are concerned that their own professional training is inadequate to provide everything that the hearing-impaired child needs. It is comforting for them to understand that they are only one, albeit important, part of the program, and that their responsibility is to enrich the child's life through group social and educational opportunities outside the home. The overall program is the ultimate responsibility of the parents and aural rehabilitation professional, with the school providing the raw material.

In-service should never be restricted to the transmission of general information about hearing loss. Such basic material should be the starting point for a targeted discussion related to the teacher's questions and observed problem areas. As the aural rehabilitation specialist presents the in-service sessions, care should be taken to avoid criticism of the program, teaching style, or curriculum. These are not the areas in which change will occur. Any programmatic concerns should have been addressed when the parents were selecting the most appropriate preschool. The question should be: Given the program as it exists, how can the management team increase the child's access to the material? Although many aspects of the teacher's presentation might be modified, it is best to target only the most glaring error, or the one that will make the most immediate difference to the hearing-impaired child. On subsequent visits, progress can be noted and new areas addressed. To reinforce discussions held at the school at the time of the observation, it is useful to provide the teacher with a written description of the positive aspects of the program and the one area in need of change.

Another aspect of in-service training is to help the teacher set appropriate expectations that account for the child's hearing loss and its effects but that use the performance of the other children as the norm. Often the teacher is unaware that the child can use anything but rudimentary speech skills, and therefore does not expect much change to occur. This low-level expectation may be reinforced by the reticence of hearing-impaired children to use their newly acquired skills in new situations. It is critical that these children demonstrate their linguistic knowledge because others' reactions are based on their perception of what the child understands and says. Careful preparation by the parent and professional before school begins can minimize this undesired behavior. Introducing the child to play groups of two, three, or four children begins to demystify the social and linguistic workings of group interaction. Adult-directed activities such as movement classes or story hour at the library can help prepare the children to take direction from adults other than their parents.

SELF-CONTAINED CLASSES

As parents explore the educational options for their preschooler, they should consider the specially designed programs for hearing-impaired children. Such classes may be part of a larger program for the hearing impaired, serving ages three to five or constitute an isolated preschool program that feeds into a variety of education programs when the children reach school age. Such center-based programs address language learning through structured, sequential steps within developmentally appropriate activities. The classes are typically five days a week to meet the intensive remedial needs of hearing-impaired preschoolers.

Characteristics of Students

Auditory Skills

The preschooler in the self-contained program typically has less developed auditory skills. Even the most rudimentary skills, such as recognizing when someone is talking, may not be at the automatic level. If the child was late-identified, giving him/her little opportunity to benefit from early intervention, amplification may be a new experience. Auditory expectations may have been minimal for such children, resulting in visual dependency.

Speech Skills

Speech delays are evident, with only approximations of words present. Situational context is required to fully understand the child's utterance. The speech production capacity of these preschoolers depends on the degree of loss, previous intervention, and demands of the home and school settings. Typically the suprasegmental aspects of speech and vowels are acquired first, with lower-frequency consonants emerging before the higher-frequency unvoiced fricatives.

Language Skills

A wide variability in language skills exists in self-contained classes. At the three-year-old level there may be several students who are in the very beginning stages of language acquisition, using primitive vocalizations combined with gesture to communicate. The same class may have students who are solidly in the one-word stage. It is a challenge for the teacher to mesh these two extremes into a group that does not penalize either. For example, the more advanced students need to be pushed to put words together, while the students at the lower end of the continuum need to develop a single-word repertoire.

Social Skills

Because of the small number of students, a self-contained class can accept a wider variability in behavior than the mainstreamed preschool. The specially trained teachers are aware of the maladaptive behaviors that can develop when children try to interpret the world through visual means. Typical behaviors include separation anxiety, selfishness, and physical expression of anger. Through the teacher's skillful shaping of their behavior over time, the students understand which behaviors are acceptable and choose to conform to them.

Parent Involvement

Most self-contained programs are five half-days a week (three hours/day = fifteen hours/week), leaving many unscheduled hours for the parents to fill. Some parents choose to provide their preschoolers with an additional learning experience in a play group/nursery school situation with normally hearing peers. Others find neighborhood social experiences to enrich their child's life. Most important is that the time spent outside of the school environment be socially and linguistically productive for the hearing-impaired child, for without this stimulation he/she will make only minimal progress.

Service Provision

Auditory Support

Self-contained classrooms have typically been designed to accommodate the listening needs of hearing-impaired children. They have sound-absorbing surfaces to reduce the noise and reverberation that interfere with speech reception. Physical modifications include ceilings that are covered with acoustic tile, floors with carpets, and walls with corkboard. Attention to location of the classroom relative to external noise from the street, playground, cafeteria, gymnasium, music room, and hall should have been given when the room was designed. Many sources of internal noise are difficult to avoid, especially in older school buildings where heating, lighting, plumbing, and wooden floors exacerbate the problem. An analysis of the listening environment is thus always in order.

Along with the effects of such physical modifications, people-generated noise is decreased since most classes have a maximum of eight children with a teacher and an assistant, compared to mainstream preschool classes with twelve to twenty children and two or three adults. The kind of noise generated by these two groups of preschool children differs greatly. The self-contained classes, certainly at the younger ages, are composed of children who are preverbal or at best newly verbal, making their verbal interaction minimal. In contrast, they are much more likely than mainstreamed children to resort to vocal/gestural means for interacting with each other. Thus the child-generated noise is likely to consist of nonspeech vocalizations, especially during the unstructured periods of the day. Conversely, in mainstream classes the highly verbal normally hearing children provide a background of conversation during unstructured activities that becomes interfering noise when the hearing-impaired child is trying to receive speech.

Teachers of hearing-impaired students are typically aware of their listening needs and employ strategies that effectively enhance speech reception in the classroom environment. The same general listening modifications described in the mainstream preschool section should be in place in these classes.

Auditory Expectations

In the self-contained environment, the demand to rely on speech input received through the auditory channel may be severely limited. Due to the classroom emphasis on compensatory visual display, demonstration, and gestural support, the child is much less likely than in a mainstream placement to depend on auditory input for understanding what is said. Although specific auditory training activities may be carried out and amplification checked daily, it is the minute-by-minute expectation that audition is important that teaches students to depend on hearing for reception and self-monitoring. Having an environment that is attuned to all aspects of sound is critical to making significant gains in auditory-linguistic development (Pollack and Ernst, 1973).

Visual Support

Self-contained classes are designed to assist the hearing-impaired student in compensating for the loss of hearing by increasing visual support. At the initial stages, this approach requires providing a heavy situational context that is obvious to the child through visual observation Concepts are demonstrated, written about, and discussed with associated pictures present. Such visual representations are presented with the speech the child hears in order to establish meaning. It is the child's task to retain the meanings of words after the visual supports have been eliminated.

Given the frequency with which such visual supports are used, it is important that the teacher be aware of their optimal use. As in the mainstream classes, the teacher should consciously shift the children's attention from the visual display and back to the face as the primary focus of the input changes.

Media

The media used in self-contained classes is usually adapted to the needs of the students. All media would include a visual component or be interpreted by the teacher, who increases their visibility by saying the words. Movies and videos with real actors are favored over those with cartoon characters, who are impossible to speechread. If cartoons are used, the teacher must interpret the action so that the children can understand the words.

Parent Involvement

Most problematic with this type of class is the noninvolvement of parents. Although the school's intent may be to keep parents informed and involved in the learning process, it is difficult, when children are transported to the school setting, to provide them with anything other than written daily reports. Parents find it difficult to translate these daily reports into home activities that reinforce and stimulate the child's learning. It may require extraordinary efforts on the part of the teacher and motivated parents to maintain the high level of interaction that occurred in the home-based parent/infant program prior to entry into preschool. Many parents express a sense of relief when their child is finally enrolled in a full-time program and someone else is "responsible" for his/her progress. To counteract this assumption of "changed responsibility," the parent must be made a partner in the educational effort, not just an informed participant. This may require that the teacher plan curricula and activities with the input of parents, giving the home activities as much importance as those that take place in school.

With equal amounts of time spent at home and school, enhancement of the home environment is a critical issue. The school personnel's interaction with the caregiver may include any of the following:

- keep home informed as to progress, problem areas, specific concepts to be addressed during the week to come; ways to stimulate these concepts in the home environment.
- get information from home regarding performance on the home assignments; on carryover of previous skills; on newly acquired information.
- get parents, in person, to demonstrate how the child is performing on a targeted skill.
- get school, in person, to demonstrate how the child is performing on a targeted skill.

It is a combination of center-based school activities and those that are most easily accomplished within home routines that provide the hearing-impaired child with the most comprehensive program. Each setting provides unique ways of stimulating and reinforcing language and speech that together contribute more to the child's learning than either would alone.

Teacher In-service

The in-service requirements of center-based teachers differ greatly from those of the mainstream early childhood teacher who is unfamiliar with hearing impairment and its sequelae. Teachers of the hearing impaired are well prepared for the communicative disruption resulting from a significant hearing loss.

Conversely, to maintain high levels of expectation these teachers need to regularly evaluate their estimation of "normal" and apply it to the progress of their students. Without such a realistic assessment of function, a common performance level appropriate for the class as a whole or the hearing-impaired children in general may be accepted. This would not be reflective of a particular child's potential for progress. It is clear that higher-than expected levels of performance can be reached with the appropriate intervention. If expectations are low for the entire class, each child in the class will be affected. Regular in-service regarding normal communication development, age-appropriate academic and social language skills, and parent/child interaction can help to maintain the skill levels of these preschool teachers.

AUDITORY MANAGEMENT

Success of an auditory management program depends on the family and professionals sharing appropriate expectations and goals. For example, it is always critical that amplification not be viewed as the solution to many of the child's language problems, but as a means of accessing the speech signal. Concerns about auditory management may reach their height in preschool years. Parents who are willing to accept slower-than-average development in their infant and toddler become more concerned about equivalent delays in their preschooler. As they see children with normal hearing displaying a large vocabulary corpus and advanced syntactic forms, families have greater difficulties coping with the less advanced skills of their child. Being cognizant of the variation in skills across children with normal hearing, and knowing the pattern of normal development of auditory, speech, and language skills, helps parents and professionals place a child's abilities in perspective and make appropriate management decisions.

Hearing Aid Evaluation (HAE)

Children in the preschool age group should not be first-time hearing aid users. Parents/caregivers will thus be familiar with amplification, how it functions, how to observe responses, how to troubleshoot it, etc. However, they may still have questions about a change in amplification and provide invaluable information that will assist the audiologist in selecting, fitting, and validating the hearing aid (Maxon and Smaldino, 1991). The purpose of hearing aid evaluations is thus to change amplification.

Preschool (three to five year-old) children have the skills to provide more specific audiological information than younger children. The audiologist may nonetheless experience some difficulty using traditional clinical techniques for selecting and fitting amplification with the three to five- year-old with hearing loss. Although these children can attend to tasks for a relatively long time and provide threshold level information, it is unlikely that they have the communicative skills to report the benefits and/or problems they are experiencing. Using techniques that are appropriate for the child's age, language level, and motor skills, it is possible to obtain frequency-specific (250 through 8000 Hz), individual-ear information. Conditioned play audiometry (CPA) procedures ensure reliable responses and maintain attention to task for relatively long test periods.

Speech audiometry results are also more specific for preschool children. Individual-ear speech recognition thresholds (SRT) (picture/object pointing or talk-back) and speech discrimination can be measured. Using picture pointing tests like the Word Intelligibility by Picture Identification—WIPI (Ross and Lerman, 1970), Northwestern University Children's Perception of Speech—NU-CHIPS (Elliot and Katz, 1980), or the Early Speech Perception Test—ESP (Moog and Geers, 1988), it is possible to conduct suprathreshold assessment of residual hearing use for speech perception. Unaided versus aided comparisons are a good tool for formal assessment of amplification benefits. Children with severe to profound hearing loss may not respond to suprathreshold speech testing because the output limits of the audiometer do not accommodate their degree of hearing loss—the sound is just not loud enough for them to perceive speech sounds.

The audiologist who is more comfortable using objective measures can use the formula-based approach to hearing aid fitting. As with the infant/toddler, differences in size and shape of the ear and its resonance characteristics must be considered in selecting appropriate electroacoustic characteristics for a preschooler. Although preschool children perform relatively well in the clinical setting, it is crucial to include observational components (home and educational setting) in their HAE. For example, although output (SSPL-90) levels can be set by using a formula-based method (Bebout, 1989; Seewald and Ross, 1988) or measuring acoustic reflex thresholds, the child's responses to loud or moderately loud sounds in the home and educational environment are the true test of tolerance.

Parent/caregiver and educational professionals' reports are also important for selecting and validating personal amplification. They will provide the audiologist with specific information that can facilitate the clinical amplification measurements and/or adjustment of electroacoustic settings. The reports from the individuals who have daily contact with the child should also include responses to speech sounds. The audiologist can use these reports to become aware of potential problems that may not be readily observable or documented during the clinical evaluation.

Since preschoolers, particularly younger ones, do not readily report benefits from and/or problems with their amplification, the amplification validation techniques described in Chapter 5 must be used. Functional gain (aided versus unaided warble tone thresholds) and suprathreshold speech perception measurements using age-appropriate techniques can be quantified in the clinic.

Although observation of the child's behaviors (speech reception, perception, production) in daily listening environments provides invaluable cues to amplification benefits, comparing the clinical and observational data can reveal the need for changes in the specific hearing aid model or its electroacoustic settings. For example, a child who does not understand the difference between "cat" and "cap" when he/she did previously may need a change in high-frequency responses. Or the child who was able to produce a difference between /b/ and /m/ and is no longer able to do so may not hear the difference because the amplification does not reproduce the acoustic information necessary to make the perceptual discrimination.

Although a child cannot report a difference in sound quality, his/her changes in speech production and/or perception will give that information to the astute parent and professional. It is also crucial that observers be aware of speech perception and production difficulties associated with listening in noise. The child who can discriminate voiced and voiceless cognates in the optimal conditions (quiet, close to the sound source, loud-enough signal) of the audiometric booth may not be able to do so when the television is on in the living room or there are several children playing together in the classroom.

The preschool hearing-impaired child may be in a formal educational setting. Therefore, amplification needs and fitting validation must take into account the various communication demands of the classroom, home, and day-care settings. These varied

Table 6.5   Some items to consider when developing the IEP for the preschool child with hearing loss.

1. Determine the appropriateness of different amplification systems for different environments.
2. Establish a daily amplification troubleshooting protocol (see Appendix for details). The responsible professional should be designated in the IEP.
3. Designate a case manager (the most knowledgeable on-site professional). This individual oversees the child's program and serves as liaison among professionals and to the parents.
4. Provide for a working relationship with the child's clinical audiologist.
5. Develop an individualized in-service program (IIP). It should cover specifics of the child's educational needs; in particular, use, maintenance, and benefits of amplification (Maxon, 1990).
6. Provide for a speech-language pathologist (when he/she is not the case manager). This professional is responsible for the child's speech perception/production and language management (Brackett, 1990).
7. Provide for parent/caregiver education programs to familiarize families with normal communication development in preschoolers and expectations specific to their child.

environments produce different listening conditions and auditory expectations. For example, although binaural hearing aids may work well when the child is at home with mother or father, the noise in the classroom may make it impossible for the child to understand the teacher's instructions. A wireless FM system may thus be a better device in the school setting.

Recommendation for special classroom amplification is dependent on careful communication among the parents, educational personnel, and clinical audiologist. It is important to determine initially if there is a need for an FM system since it is not always the amplification of choice in preschool. When an FM is appropriate, the specific make, model, and settings should be determined by taking into account the child's hearing loss, the demands of the educational setting, and the expectations of the school personnel.

In the mainstream preschool, each activity should be analyzed to determine when an FM unit could be used appropriately to enhance teacher/student communication. If there is little teacher-directed activity such as circle time, songs, and stories, the child may perform better with his/her personal amplification. For the mainstreamed or self-contained class in which teacher-directed instruction occurs during much of the day, an FM unit would ensure optimal reception of speech input.

Troubleshooting

The daily troubleshooting protocol presented in the Appendix can be adapted to meet the needs of the preschooler. Parents/caregivers and educational personnel may benefit from in-service training that emphasizes the need for such a trouble-shooting program and updates them on any new skills they may need to conduct it. For example, when the child is an FM user, troubleshooting must include checking the microphone/transmitter.

The preschooler's IEP should have specific goals and objectives related to the various aspects of auditory management. The items presented in Table 6.5 should be considered for all children and incorporated as necessary.

SUMMARY

Children three to five years of age need contact with adults and peers outside of the home environment. This broadening of life experience presents a challenge for the aural rehabilitation specialist, the parent, and the child. The selection of an educational setting that will meet the child's unique needs requires careful consideration of child, parent, and school factors.

References

Bebout, J. (1989). Pediatric hearing aid fitting: A practical overview. *Hearing Journal* 42, 8, 13-20.

Brackett, D. (1990). Developing an individualized educational program for the mainstreamed hearing-impaired student. In M. Ross (Ed.) *Hearing-Impaired Children in the Mainstream*. Parkton, MD: York Press. (pp 81-94).

Elliot, L. & Katz, D. (1980). *Development of a New Children's Test of Speech Discrimination*. St. Louis, MO; Auditec.

Maxon, A.B. (1990). Implementing an in-service training program. In M. Ross (Ed.) *Hearing-Impaired Children in the Mainstream*. Parkton, MD: York Press. (pp 257-274).

Maxon, A.B. & Smaldino, J. (1991). Hearing aid management for children. *Seminars in Hearing*.

Moog, J. & Geers, A. (1988). *Early Speech Perception Test*. St. Louis, MO: Central Institute for the Deaf.

Pollack, D. & Ernst, M. (1973). Don't set limits: Expectations for preschool children. In W.H. Northcott (Ed.) *The Hearing Impaired Child in the Regular Classroom: Preschool, Primary, and Secondary Years*. Washington, DC: A.G. Bell Association.

Ross, M. & Lerman, J.W. (1970). A picture identification test for hearing impaired children. *Journal of Speech and Hearing Research* 13, 44-53.

Seewald, R.C. & Ross, M. (1988). Amplification for the young hearing impaired child. In M. Pollack (Ed.) *Amplification for the Hearing Impaired*, New York, NY. Grume and Stratton, (pp. 213-267).

7

Programming: School-age (6–21 years)

INTRODUCTION

Social and academic experiences frame a student's school life. Often professionals concentrate primarily on the academic aspects of the school experience and the academic skills needed to function in that environment. However, the actual time spent in social interaction during the school day is approximately equal to that spent in classroom learning. It is therefore important to consider both the social and academic ramifications of a particular placement, before initially selecting the placement and regularly during the student's school career.

Academic lessons place the child in a structured teacher-directed situation where his/her language inadequacies are most apparent. The teacher chooses the topics for discussion, the language used for the discussion, and the manner of assessing learning. The child adopts the role of recipient and respondent to the teacher's academic input. Academic learning depends on reading, a language-based skill. Written language transmits the student's knowledge on exams and through expository and creative writing.

It is in the social venues that the hearing-impaired student competes on the most equal footing with peers. During social interactions the topic for discussion is often directly related to the social milieu of the moment and can be initiated by any member of the group, including the hearing-impaired student. The conversational volleys are typically short, with the purpose of establishing camaraderie and joint agreement, not transmitting information. Knowing what to say, how to say it, and how to behave are skills that are critical to the child's success in any school program.

PROGRAMMING DECISIONS

If it is difficult to predict function from the audiogram of a newly identified infant, it is impossible to do so with hearing-impaired children who are school age. They have management and family histories that compound the effect of the hearing loss, resulting in enormous variability in their skill development.

There will be a group of children for whom a placement decision needs to be made because their preschool program was free standing and did not directly feed into an existing school program. There will also be parents who believe that their children have extracted as much benefit as possible from the program at the preschool level and desire a change for the school years. Often it takes a parent to "rock the boat" before changes occur.

Although more options are available at the elementary age level, most severely and profoundly hearing-impaired children will continue in the school-aged version of their parent/infant programs. In large regionalized programs the child may have the option of being totally self-contained, or mainstreamed for social and/or academic reasons. In more isolated regions of the country, the child's program may be determined by the availability of special education personnel trained to work with hearing-impaired students. The selection of either a self-contained or a mainstreamed educational setting requires the careful consideration of its social and academic demands.

The placement decision should be made based on whether the student can potentially learn more in a self-contained social, communicative, and academic environment or in a highly verbal, competitive, mainstream class. How much can potentially be learned in any setting is difficult to determine. It is clear that every normally hearing child who sits in a regular education classroom does not learn all the material that is presented by the teacher. In fact, the actual amount of information learned and retained from a single "lecture" may be small. However, the normally hearing student with age-appropriate language skills can understand the words that are said and learn the concepts when attending to the teacher. The hearing-impaired student is at a disadvantage compared to his/her normally hearing peers since he/she enters the mainstream classroom with an underdeveloped linguistic foundation. When hearing-impaired students enter such a highly verbal situation their job is twofold: comprehending the words and sentences used to transmit the concepts and learning the concepts themselves. These two tasks occupy all of the child's attention, leaving little free time to daydream or be inattentive. If their attention wanders they usually sacrifice one of these two primary aspects of learning.

Conversely, the hearing-impaired student in the self-contained class can understand and learn material as a result of the appropriate teaching style and simplified language used. Ease of learning is not the only criterion to be considered however. In determining if a self-contained class is appropriate, the critical factor is the actual grade level and complexity of the lessons. The teacher of hearing-impaired students typically adapts the language level to the majority of the children in the class. Children who are functioning at either end of the academic performance continuum therefore have to settle for learning material that is presented either above or below their skill level (not unlike the situation that faces some normally hearing children in regular classes). Although it may be advantageous for the child at the lower end of the continuum to be exposed to and possibly reach the level of the majority, a self-contained placement has a negative effect on the student at the upper margin.

The question remains, Is the age-appropriate information that is only partially understood and learned in the mainstream more, less, or equivalent to the adapted information learned in the self-contained class? This question needs to be asked at regular intervals in the child's school career. If the answer favors the self-contained class, the child educated in the mainstream requires a change of placement. If it seems that the student can receive an equal amount of information in the mainstream setting, then plans should be made to place the child in the least restrictive environment possible.

School professionals who have limited experience with managing the educational needs of hearing-impaired students propose "being with one's own kind" as a rationale for a self-contained placement. Although having the support and understanding of a peer group with a similar handicapping condition is valuable, it should be an extenuating factor rather than the main reason for an educational placement. If the child finds him/herself in an educational environment in which no other hearing-impaired students are present, support staff (teachers of the hearing impaired, speech-language pathologists, audiologists) should orchestrate contacts with other hearing-impaired children. As long as the child feels socially integrated, the placement meets his/her social needs. This situation differs from the child who feels socially isolated in a mainstream environment and requests a change in placement so that he/she can belong to a group.

MAINSTREAM OPTION

Mainstream education includes any educational situation in which the student has contact with nonhearing-impaired peers. Ross, Brackett and Maxon (1991) fully describe the evaluation and management of this population. The contact includes interactions in the social and academic venues. Full mainstreaming is defined as educational programming in which the student receives all of his/her education in the regular classroom. All remedial services are provided outside of the classroom and support the regular education program. Partial mainstreaming occurs when the student has some but not all of his/her education with normally hearing students. The remainder of the educational program takes place in the special education classroom with hearing-impaired peers. When all academic subjects are carried out in the special education classes yet opportunities exist for social contact with normally hearing peers, the program is defined as social mainstreaming. In this book, social mainstreaming will be addressed under self-contained classes even though opportunities exist for interacting with normally hearing peers during nonacademic and nonschool activities.

Well-intentioned educators and parents underutilize mainstream classes as a placement for severely and profoundly hearing-impaired children with the requisite entry skills. This placement should be selected not only when other specialized educational services are absent, but for what it can offer, i.e., a rich auditory verbal environment, normal expectations, and good speech models. Mainstreaming should be actively considered as a choice as long as the student has the entry skills to compete with normally hearing peers.

Characteristics of Setting

The mainstreamed learning environment contains many positive as well as negative features, all of which should be considered. Such features need to be weighed against each other to determine if the negative ones will interfere with learning or if they can be managed by the student. The three most important features are as follows:

Rich auditory verbal environment
Typical classrooms contain many opportunities for the child to listen to sound, both speech and noise, generated by students. Not all of this sound is purposeful. Although the speech used during peer-to-peer interaction or teacher/child contacts is productive, much of the noise generated by the students as they move furniture, slam books, or shuffle papers needs to be ignored. Normally hearing students are able to separate the pertinent speech from the more diffuse noise that threatens to cover up the meaningful elements. Hearing-impaired students are unable to make this distinction, causing them to work especially hard to perceive the speech within a prominent background of interfering noise. The auditory system is actively stimulated in this environment.

Poor acoustic environment
To complicate matters, the acoustic characteristics of untreated mainstream classrooms increase the intensity and continuation of noise. Hard surfaces, utilized in public spaces because they are easy to clean, perpetuate the louder elements of speech long after the original signal has diminished. This reverberated sound interferes with the perception of the primary speech signal.

Teachers inexperienced with hearing-impaired children
Regular educators are trained to present the curriculum to normally hearing children in a stimulating, effective manner. Such teachers bring a unique perspective to the education of hearing-impaired children. They expect any child who is present in the classroom to exhibit normal social, academic, and communicative behaviors. The hearing-impaired student is expected to conform to the "normal" standard. Reaching this goal is possible for hearing-impaired students who possess appropriate entry skills.

Regular education teachers have typically neither received any information on the learning needs of hearing-impaired students during their coursework nor experienced an equivalent educational challenge previously in their careers. Their intent and willingness to help may be genuine, but their inexperience with hearing-impaired children can be counterproductive unless in-service training is provided.

Characteristics of Students

The child's success in a mainstreamed setting hinges on the presence or absence of particular personality traits, communication abilities, and academic skills. Mainstreaming assumes that the child can communicate effectively with peers and adults, can learn from normal behavioral models, and has strong self-esteem and motivation to learn.

In order to benefit from such an academically stimulating environment, the student must possess sufficient communication skills to perform both the oral and written work of the classroom and to interact with peers and adults. Placement in a mainstreamed setting assumes that the child has the social and academic skills to compete with his/her normally hearing classmates. Contact with normally hearing peers places certain demands on the child. The teacher expects the child to understand the lecture and what is read, and to respond appropriately in speech and writing.

The hearing-impaired student who is unable to interact socially with normally hearing peers will have difficulty in successfully maintaining the mainstream placement. Social skills must mirror those of normally hearing classmates, particularly in regard to interaction style, interests, independence, and sexual maturity. The situation of the socially isolated student is analogous to that of the gifted child who enters high school four to five years before his/her same-aged peers—the only area in common with his/her classmates is the academic work itself. Although the hearing-impaired student is chronologically the same age as his/her classmates, social immaturity may place him/her out of the mainstream.

Auditory Skills

Candidates for a mainstreamed placement are often children with the lesser degrees of hearing loss or the fortunate severely or profoundly impaired children who have benefited from very early intervention and an aggressive amplification fitting/use program (Davis and Hardick, 1981). These students are dependent on auditory input for receiving the speech of others and monitoring their own speech productions (Northcott, 1973).

Brackett and Maxon (1986) describe the auditory function and dependence of a group of fully mainstreamed children. The average hearing loss was 65dB HL with a range from 0 (unilateral loss) to 110dB. A comparison of the average auditory-only and auditory-visual word recognition scores demonstrates the dependence on auditory information for this group.

Speech Intelligibility

Speech intelligibility must be sufficient for sending a message via spoken language that can be understood by normally hearing peers and adults. This requirement in no way implies that the articulation, voice, intonation, pitch, and rhythm of mainstreamed students will be without effects from the hearing loss, but indicates only that their speech must be intelligible. Since such students are dependent on their hearing, their speech production errors often reflect speech perception abilities. Errors are typically made on speech sounds that differ only according to place of articulation, e.g., /k/ versus /t/, since the acoustic energy required to differentiate between them is carried in the high frequencies, an area of the speech spectrum that is least accessible to hearing-impaired children.

Language Level

Comprehension and production of spoken language must be adequate for understanding the messages of both peers and adults, and for putting words together in a way that clearly codes the intended message. Language skills need to be within the range exhibited by other members of the class into which the child is placed. This does not mean that all aspects of language will be equally developed. Often students will have sufficient social grammar to communicate in nonstructured social activities but have difficulty when confronted with the nonconversational style of written language. Typical errors of school-age hearing-impaired children include inadequate vocabulary, omission of verb endings, and simplified syntax, although a wide range of skills is exhibited by children in mainstream settings (Maxon and Brackett, 1987; Brackett and Maxon, 1986).

Academic Skills

Academic skills should also be compatible with existing levels in the regular classroom (Northcott, 1973). Ideally the child will function somewhere in the middle of the class in some or all of the academic subjects. With most mainstream classes having performance levels that vary by as much as one to two years around the actual grade level, it should be possible to accommodate the differing needs of these hearing-impaired students. Mainstreamed students typically demonstrate the greatest academic deficiencies in language-based subjects such as language arts, reading, or other subjects that require extensive reading to convey content (social studies, science). Subjects such as math usually show these students at their best.

Social Skills

As long as the student desires to be part of a group he/she is likely to learn from peer models. It requires a strong sense of self-worth to be the only student with an obvious "difference" in a class or school. Students should demonstrate age-appropriate classroom and conversational interaction skills and exhibit a strong self-concept.

Parental Involvement

As in the preschool years, strong parental support and involvement is required when the child is educated in a mainstreamed environment. With teachers who are inexperienced in presenting the curriculum to hearing-impaired students and the presence of poor acoustic conditions, parents need to support the efforts of the regular educator by providing home reinforcement.

Social and Academic Expectations in Mainstream Settings

An examination of the social and academic expectations for normally hearing children in regular education provides insight into areas of potential disruption for the mainstreamed hearing-impaired student.

Elementary (5–10 years)

The hearing-impaired child may still be adjusting to a large class size. If this is a first mainstream experience the child may need a long adjustment period to modify his/her behaviors to accommodate large-group demands. A student-teacher ratio of 6:2 in self-contained or preschool programs encourages more direct teacher contact than does the typical classroom ratio of 25:1. The higher student-teacher ratio forces the child to be independent. Self-motivation thus plays a large role in how successfully the child handles such a placement. In the regular education class, the hearing-impaired child must independently complete seatwork and remain attentive to the lecture. For the child recently mainstreamed from a self-contained setting, such self-directed skills may be lacking.

It is impossible in a mainstream setting for a regular classroom teacher to wait for each of the twenty-five students to master the content of the lesson before moving on to new material. Instead, the teacher introduces new concepts from the curriculum at regular short intervals. The expectation is that the students will make the effort to learn the material by attending to lectures and completing the required paperwork. The redundancy present in the self-contained class is noticeably absent. Since the teacher cannot check on every aspect of each child's work, the hearing-impaired child must be motivated not only to learn the material, but also to ask for assistance when needed.

Competition is an accepted aspect of regular education programs, resulting from the grading system used. By first grade, teachers indicate right and wrong answers and judge the child's written work accordingly. Thus competition builds among students who vie for the best grades. If such grades are achievable by the hearing-impaired child the competition can have a positive effect. However, for the child who is working to potential but cannot attain grades consistent with the best students in the class, competition only creates frustration. The hearing-impaired child who was previously educated in a self-contained class may be unprepared for this competitive experience due to the typically ungraded nature of special education.

When twenty-five children are grouped in a class, it is typical that subgroups form based on interests, status, etc. These subgroups are flexible and change according to the characteristics of the children included. The hearing-impaired child must learn how to enter and exit these groups effectively. This requires knowledge of the commonalities that join the group and techniques for accessing them. Many newly mainstreamed hearing-impaired children will have little experience with subgroup formation since the groups in the self-contained setting are small (six children) and few child-initiated activities are included in the day.

Junior High School (11–13 years)

The preadolescent period is difficult for hearing-impaired children. Not only do they have to adjust to the changing demands of the academic setting, but they must also contend with increased social pressures.

Departmentalized teaching forces hearing-impaired children to adjust to multiple teachers' speech and teaching style. Their success or failure in a subject area may be due to the teacher's understanding of the requisite classroom modifications. Not only the presentation styles are different but also the expectations and demands. Hearing-impaired students may be unaware of the adjustments required to learn from multiple teachers, since in their past educational experience the educators adjusted their interactions to the needs of the student. In junior high school, children are expected to adapt to the teachers.

Class placement for middle school or junior high school students depends on their learning potential and/or class performance. Skillstreaming may be a new concept for the hearing-impaired child. In special education, classes are typically composed of same-aged children with similar handicapping conditions, and the actual skill level of the individual children may vary greatly.

The homogeneous grouping of the junior high school mainstreamed classes can have both positive and negative effects on the students. They may be tracked into a language arts/English class with children who exhibit similar performance profiles in language-based subjects (the hearing-impaired child's most deficient area). The different interests, limited curiosity, and lack of motivation of their skill-matched classmates often interferes, however, with the hearing-impaired students' desire and potential to learn. It is the hearing-impaired students' lack of linguistic experience and competence that affects their performance, rather than the behavioral or motivational issues that may be the underlying difficulty for the normally hearing students in the class. It may, however, be possible through negotiation to track the hearing-impaired child at a level slightly higher than the one at which he/she is performing, using potential to learn as the rationale.

The more competent students may find themselves in a highly competitive learning environment with other students having relatively matched skills and motivation. Thus a situation in which they could have excelled is converted to one in which they must fight to be noticed. Usually such problems of tracking are less evident in nonlanguage-based subjects, in which the child's abilities are most evident.

The middle school/junior high experience also introduces new school routines that may tax the ability of the hearing-impaired student. Learning to use the library, synthesize information, and write an expository treatise are introduced at this age so that mastery can occur by high school. These skills require a level of language expertise that is difficult for many hearing-impaired children to attain.

Most obvious are the social changes that occur at this age. Parental influence decreases with the increase in peer pressure to conform. Choosing between the values of parents and those of peers places the child in a difficult position. The exposure to different beliefs and life-styles can be broadening since it represents "the real world." However, children are easily frightened when expected to deal with unfamiliar situations for which they lack the strategies for effective resolution. If moral development has been intense it is likely that at this point the child will remain under the parents' direction (often reluctantly). The more homogeneous the community and school, the more likely it is that children with the same level of moral development will adhere to their parents' teaching. Due to the racial, ethnic, and socioeconomic mix of most public schools, however, few families have such a simple situation to work with (unless a parochial or private school has been selected).

During adolescence, increased mobility physically distances the child from the nuclear family. Most children request permission to be independently mobile. No longer is it appropriate for parents to escort the child to and from activities. Instead, groups of similarly aged children often go and return from activities unchaperoned. Lack of independence and/or parental overprotectiveness can lead to lack of mobility and peer disapproval for the child.

Interest in the opposite sex and concern about one's external appearance emerges at this age level. Noticing and emulating the clothing and behavior of a selected peer group becomes a paramount concern. Differences are noticed, commented upon, and often become the basis of rejection for group membership. For example, the need to wear an FM unit or visible hearing aids signals a difference.

For the parent of the hearing-impaired child, it is a time of letting go, of loosening control over the child's social interactions. It is typical for the parent to prolong the dependence of early childhood since it includes a "protective" feature. But by continuing to have a parent-directed life, the hearing-impaired child will have little opportunity to acquire the skills for making decisions.

For the obviously hearing-impaired student wearing visible amplification, this period of conformity is often difficult. There is a need to continually prove his/her worth as a group member to avoid rejection. To have a hearing-impaired student as a member of a group causes all members to justify their choice. If the hearing-impaired student displays behavior that attracts attention, his/her welcome as a group member is diminished. Conversely, if after being conditionally accepted in the group the student brings acceptable attention to it (winning awards, excelling in athletics, demonstrating a creative talent), then continued group membership is assured.

Male-female relationships at this age are typically one-sided and group-related. Contact with the opposite sex thus remains positive as long as group membership continues. Sexual attraction stimulates two opposing kinds of behavior. Initially, the child desperately seeks to be viewed as a valued group member by the chosen opposite-sex person. Simultaneously the desire to be noticed is strong but difficult to satisfy in a highly conforming group. For example, it is hard to distinguish female teens who share group membership since they adopt similar hair styles, clothing, and mannerisms.

Most hearing-impaired students struggle with their group and opposite-sex relationships beginning in this preteen era and continuing through high school. It is easy to blame the hearing loss and wearing hearing aids for all the overwhelming social issues that arise during this period, when in reality at least some of the problems can be attributed to age. Parents may find that their own long-standing fears about "social acceptance" reappear, making it difficult to provide the support that the child needs to adjust to developmental changes. If a child laments about lack of friends, female or male, parents may convey through body language and facial expression that they feel sorry for the child even though the actual words said are supportive, thereby communicating a mixed message.

High School (14–18 years)

Students are grouped academically, according to ability, being judged on their performance during in-class discussions as well as through written papers and tests. Thinking rather than the regurgitation of facts is encouraged in the higher-tracked classes. The hearing-impaired student in these classes is forced to use abstract thinking and inference, a demonstrated area of weakness, in academic interactions. Accordingly, support services should focus on helping such students write and discuss the abstract ideas incorporated in mainstream high school classes.

The lower tracks are oriented toward vocational training, with an option of post-secondary training. Many hearing-impaired students are directed toward these tracks by the kind and quality of education they receive. For example, without college preparatory courses they are at a disadvantage when competing with their peers on the SAT. Many students opt for receiving their postsecondary education in colleges that have modified curricula or adaptations to facilitate classroom communication.

At this age normally hearing students are beginning to set their sights to the future. They worry about what will happen to them next in their lives, what their future employment possibilities include, whether their teen relationships will persist in the postsecondary years. The social insecurity of this period is highly manifest. Students live for each day without considering the long-term effects of their actions. Academically, choices in coursework are related to future career goals. Achieving passing grades begins to take on new meaning as postsecondary education looms on the horizon. Hearing-impaired adolescents are equally concerned about their futures, which hold additional uncertainties. Their decisions regarding social and academic identity groups impact on their choices of college, training program, and profession.

High school represents a time when social and academic demands must be balanced to produce well-adjusted students able to achieve their potential. Peer pressure remains strong, but individualistic traits also begin to emerge. Social groupings are made along a variety of parameters: academic, interest, ethnicity. Hearing-impaired students, who suffered from being different during the junior high period, begin to establish an identity group, either normally hearing or hearing impaired. As long as the student has something to offer to a group (sports ability, art talent), obvious differences (use of hearing aids, speech sound distortions) may be overlooked in favor of group acceptance. Male-female attraction is an additional issue since one's acceptance often depends on the acceptability of the partner. As long as individual differences are accepted, hearing-impaired students can gain acceptance as an opposite-sex partner.

Time spent away from the family continues to increase, with outside influences having potentially dramatic impact. Although moral behavior was established earlier, students are now faced with the choice of acting in accordance with family morality or feeling "guilty" about their behavior. Parents of hearing-impaired students have to be confident that they have established a strong moral base in the early years that will control the student's behavior when he/she is with others. Proper preparation is critical for the parents and child to feel confident that the child will know what to do when confronted with the unfamiliar or unknown.

Service Provision

Given the academic and social demands in the mainstream, it will be necessary to assist the hearing-impaired student in maintaining grade-level academic achievement and age-level communication/social skills.

Auditory Learning
Instead of performing listening training as a separate activity, the speech-language pathologist should incorporate listening into all aspects of the remedial program by presenting vocabulary, grammar, and syntax without speechreading cues. Speech correction is most effective when the auditory feedback system is exploited for monitoring speech. A coordinated program that integrates language, speech, and listening goals and relates to both academic and social aspects of the child's life is most effective (Erber, 1982).

In mainstream classes, reduced full-face speechreading cues forces reliance on aided residual hearing for receiving the teacher's speech. Regular education teachers often talk and write on the board simultaneously, hold objects or papers in front of the face, or point at a key word on the board while lecturing. The student who has the ability to understand speech through auditory-only input or to piece together the incomplete message will have a distinct advantage. The rich auditory conditions of the mainstream classroom provide many opportunities for "auditory-based learning" to take place. Unlike the teacher of a self-contained class, however, the regular educator will be unaware of the student's day-to-day auditory functioning as long as he/she "appears" to hear.

Since school is a time when it is important for the child to have access to the full speech signal, every effort should be made to enhance the auditory and visual aspects of the teacher's presentation. Keeping the teacher's face visible during all instruction is a primary focus of any in-service sessions. Instead of memorizing the typical situations that reduce face visibility, the teacher needs only to remember that his/her face must be in full sight of the hearing-impaired student whenever spoken information is presented to the class.

Other visual support in the form of written words on the board, outlines, maps, objects, or gesture all reinforce the words being said. The list below describes the modifications that the classroom teacher can implement to facilitate learning for all the children in the class.

Provide optimal seating to allow child full visual access to teacher.

Use FM to achieve improved reception of the primary sound source in typical classroom noise.

Maintain full view of teacher's face during presentation of lessons. Avoid speaking with back turned to class.

Use written support in the form of outlines, assignments, key words, and change in topic.

Use additional visual aids/media to supplement spoken information in lessons.

Assign a buddy/classmate who can help maintain child's attention to task.

Engage a notetaker to write down pertinent information discussed by class members or included in lecture, leaving the hearing-impaired child free to maintain visual contact with the speaker.

Preview and review of content material in academic support sessions.

Install sound-absorbing surfaces (carpeting, corkboard) to improve the signal-to-noise ratio.

Check personal and classroom amplification daily. Classroom teacher should have a wand and extra cord and batteries provided by the family and/or rehabilitation personnel.

Coordinate closely with special education staff to ensure mastery of academic material.

Avoid simultaneously speaking and calling attention to a visual aid to allow student full access to speechreading clues and visual display.

Language Level

Every interaction that the hearing-impaired student has with the teacher or other students in the mainstream represents an opportunity to learn and refine his/her language system. If the student receives academic support, language learning also occurs when the tutor explains concepts and previews/reviews classroom lessons. Although exposure to new forms, vocabulary, and information in the classroom is beneficial to language learning, the classroom teacher does not teach language development as a subject area, but uses language arts as a vehicle for learning about the grammatical structure of English.

Specific vocabulary, form, and usage deficits identified during the comprehensive communication evaluation are addressed during the individual speech/language therapy. Whenever possible the information included in the classroom lessons should be used as stimuli for the language sessions. To be effectively integrated into all aspects of the mainstream setting, students need special instruction in the appropriate use of language in specific social situations.

Speech Intelligibility

Speech production remediation is conducted outside of the classroom during individually scheduled sessions. To maximally utilize time out of the classroom, speech targets can be incorporated into the language development portion of the session rather than addressed separately. Effective speech management for the school-age child demands that classroom vocabulary and concepts be used as stimuli for the speech production exercises. Since a classroom teacher can provide only rudimentary monitoring of the speech targets, the student must be able to self-correct the errors within the session and generalize them to other situations. Automatic usage outside of the structured sessions remains the responsibility of the parent and child.

Academic Skills

The teacher in the regular education classroom follows a planned curriculum, moving to new topics according to a fixed schedule. For mastery of this fast-paced material to occur, the hearing-impaired student may require more repetition than is possible in the classroom.

A supplemental academic support program (tutoring, resource room) familiarizes the student with classroom concepts prior to a lesson and reinforces them at regular intervals in the days following it. Instead of using a separate curriculum, this support service supplements the information presented during classroom lectures, thus enhancing the educational process. Other classroom supports include an interpreter (sign, oral, or cued speech) and a notetaker.

Social Skills

It is the parents' responsibility to socialize their children to behavior appropriate for the family's community. Part of the socialization process includes learning what to say in specific situations and ways of adapting communication to the listener. By orchestrating social contacts, parents can afford children opportunities to use skills and receive feedback about them.

Therapeutic intervention may be required if the student enters the mainstream setting without acceptable social behaviors. Since hearing-impaired students want to be accepted by their peers, often an explanation of their acts viewed as deviant by others can diminish their use. These students typically lack an understanding of subtle humor, friendly name calling, idiomatic expressions, and figurative language. They may misunderstand an offhand comment and be offended by it. Intervention may also focus on effective styles of presenting answers, arguing, and negotiating in spoken and written language.

Parent Involvement

Parents need to be active participants in the process for effective mainstreaming to occur. During the school years, parents reinforce classroom learning by monitoring homework, socializing the child to acceptable community standards, and providing learning experiences to supplement classroom curriculum.

The most successful children have parents who recognize what is expected of the student, monitor learning through homework assignments, and encourage independence and responsibility. Two scenarios that should be avoided are as follows: (1) the parent who is overly involved in the day-to-day workings of the class, insisting on daily calls from the teacher regarding the student's functioning; (2) the parent who rarely has contact with the teacher except when problems have emerged in the classroom and the teacher requests a meeting. Both of these parenting styles dilute the student's ability to function independently.

SELF-CONTAINED OPTIONS

Self-contained classes are a viable option for many severely and profoundly hearing-impaired children. These classes can be categorized by location (day classes in public schools, residential schools for the deaf), or by the amount of contact with normally hearing students (residential—none; day classes—nonacademic interaction).

Day Classes

Public School

These programs are designed to optimize social contact with normally hearing peers without sacrificing the specially modified academic curriculum. The potential for social interaction occurs in the nonacademic time periods such as lunch and recess, or in the "specials" — music, gym, art, home economics or industrial arts. Although this placement has many social and communication benefits for the hearing-impaired child, it has the negative effect of emphasizing the differences between the two groups of children. The discrepancy between their academic, social, and communicative skills is made evident whenever the two groups interact. To effectively utilize the potential of housing this class in a building with normally hearing children, the special education teacher has to make a conscious attempt to integrate his/her students into school activities—otherwise the class becomes an entity unto itself, gaining none of the benefits of being housed with normally hearing students.

Day class attendance allows children to live at home and develop a sense of self within their community. It is especially beneficial to the child if family/child communication is effective and the child is considered a part of the family. Davis and Hardick (1981) describe the increased independence that is possible when the child remains a functioning member of his/her home community.

School for the Deaf

In recent years, schools for the deaf have refocused their curricula to reflect the trend toward nonresidential education for hearing-impaired children. Day students predominate in such a segregated setting. Although its academic demands may be similar to those of a day class housed in a regular school, a school for the deaf cannot replicate social interactions with normally hearing students. If the student lives at home, the parents become responsible for orchestrating the social interactions, such as boy scouts or town sports, that assist him/her in learning acceptable behaviors.

Residential

For a small number of hearing-impaired students, a residential school for the deaf represents the only avenue to quality education. This option is chosen when the student resides in a geographical area that lacks the type of education required, or when the nearest day program is not within an hour commuting distance. To maintain family ties, the student goes home each weekend if possible. Thus residential students learn to adapt to the demands of two environments, one modified to meet the needs of the hearing-impaired, and the other expecting mainstream social skills to be used. For those students who live at extended distances, social and recreational activities at the school fill the weekend. The house parents become surrogate family for such residential students. All social, recreational, and academic contact is with other hearing-impaired students and there is minimal interaction with normally hearing individuals.

A residential option is also selected when the student requires a controlled living environment due to behavioral/emotional problems or a disruptive home environment. If the student demonstrates asocial behaviors, such as stealing, pyromania, or fighting, in a less restricted setting and all attempts at correcting them have failed, he/she may need a placement in which activity can be closely monitored. A dysfunctional home can also place the student at risk for poor school attendance as well as other manifestations of neglect. The residential setting provides the structure, motivation, and interest that is lacking for children when parents or caregivers cannot manage the situation. In the supportive atmosphere provided by teachers and dorm parents, such children can attain their potential and establish self-esteem and self-worth.

Residential students are grouped with day-program students during the academic day, but interaction during after-school and weekend activities is limited to a subgroup of dorm students. The dorm parents and school staff are responsible for "socializing" the residential students through typical family-oriented activities. Learning to share, contributing in a group, obeying adults, and having responsibilities are skills that "normalize" the child as a social being.

Characteristics of Setting

The self-contained environment is a highly adapted environment designed to meet the listening, communication, and academic needs of selected hearing-impaired students. These modifications (listed below) are ideal for the student who requires an adapted curriculum and teaching style in order to learn.

Controlled language input
The teacher of the hearing impaired adapts the classroom language to present the subject matter at level understood by the students. Science, social studies, and mathematics may contain content similar to the regular classroom, but the language is simplified to accommodate the students' reduced language competency. The texts are high interest and low vocabulary to ensure that the concepts are learned even if the details are discounted. This approach is effective for the student who enters the educational setting with deficient vocabulary and syntax.

Structured sequential language curriculum
In addition to using teacher input that is more repetitious and less complex syntactically and lexically, the self-contained class has a built-in language curriculum designed to facilitate language growth. Usually the form and content of the English language is taught through small sequential steps using spoken and written stimuli. It remains a subject area throughout the child's school years or until the rudiments are mastered.

Protected academic and social environment
The self-contained environment provides security for the student who lacks the linguistic competence to compete on equal footing with normally hearing peers. The highly competitive character of the regular classroom is absent. Each student's strengths and weaknesses are recognized and accepted so that growth is fostered in all areas without damage to self-esteem. In a small class, the teacher is more likely to provide multiple repetitions, to proceed at a slower pace, and to accept marginal social behaviors.

Modified acoustic environments
It is expected that self-contained classrooms will be specifically adapted to meet the auditory and visual learning needs of the hearing-impaired student. Carpeting, curtains, and acoustic ceiling tile absorb sound and allow the primary speech signal to be received without the interference of reverberated noise. Group teaching areas are designed so that the students are not looking into glare from the window as they attend to the teacher.

Experienced teachers

Self-contained classes are staffed with teachers who are knowledgeable about hearing impairment, its effects, and management strategies. They are aware of the changes in teaching style that facilitate learning, such as allowing full visual access, decreasing distance between teacher and students, and providing visual support and demonstration for the lecture.

Characteristics of Students

These are children who require the specific features of the self-contained class and are not just placed there because they have a hearing loss. The rationale for placement must be based on the need for controlled language input, structured sequential language curriculum, and a protected academic and social environment. Candidates for the self-contained classes are characterized by their competence in the following areas:

Auditory Skills

Paul and Quigley (1990) report that students in self-contained classes have a greatly reduced amplification usage rate (30%) compared to students educated in mainstreamed classes (78%). Whether the low rate of usage is due to the lack of demands in the classroom or modification of teacher demands based on the students' limited use is impossible to determine.

It is clear that an environment that provides supplementary visual input during all activities does not encourage use of hearing. Teachers who flick the lights on, touch the students, or stamp their feet to gain attention are conveying the message that using visual, tactile, or vibrotactile input is sufficient. It is not surprising that these students are reluctant to wear visible amplification when its value appears limited.

Speech Intelligibility

The speech intelligibility of self-contained students varies according to the degree of loss, the frequency and quality of intervention, and the demand for speech in the classroom environment. They typically exhibit multiple articulation errors and omissions, disruption in stress and intonation, and pitch instability and elevation. This error pattern is not surprising since they are exposed to the deficient speech of their peers six hours per day, in addition to not using their hearing for monitoring their own speech productions. The greatest negative impact on speech production is, however, the low expectations of teachers, rehabilitation providers, and parents.

Language Level

Students in this setting typically exhibit significant language delays relative to their same-aged normally hearing peers. Specific delays in vocabulary, grammar, and syntax make it difficult for these children to develop age-appropriate written/read language. Often they have learned language through written reinforcement and thus exhibit better written than spoken language.

Academic Skills

The performance level of these students typically falls one and one-half to two years below expected grade level, with language-based subjects showing the greatest delays. It is this delay and their need for intensive, structured teaching that make these students candidates for the self-contained setting.

Social Skills

Due to the protected nature of the environment, the students in self-contained placements tend to develop coping and problem-solving strategies later than their peers. Since adults often intervene in disputes, in class preparation, and in social interactions, it takes longer for the student to acquire self-help skills. Parents may be pleased that their children are enrolled in the protective cocoon of the self-contained class since it prevents them from being exposed to the troubles of the "real" world. However, prolonged immaturity results when the parents accept behavior appropriate for much younger children.

Parent Involvement

Many of the parents' responsibilities are assumed by the classroom teacher when the student is enrolled in a self-contained class. The reinforcement of classroom concepts is included in each activity. Since the student is home for only part of the day, parent involvement must by necessity be more limited. Parental involvement is severely restricted in residential settings, with any out-of-class reinforcement provided by school staff.

Social and Academic Aspects of Self-contained Classes

The positive and negative aspects of a self-contained placement are described below according to age.

Elementary (5–10 years)

The small class size ensures more one-to-one contact than is possible in classes with normally hearing children. Individualized attention allows the student to proceed at his/her own rate through a sequential pattern of language and content material. This positive aspect is counteracted by dependence on the adult for assistance. This dependence can be diminished by gradually reducing the amount of help provided and insisting on maximum effort by the child before the request for help is made.

Self-contained programs are teacher-directed with attention to the teacher demanded during "lecture" times. If the child's attention wanders, the teacher calls his/her name, or will even stop talking until all eyes are appropriately directed. Seatwork is conducted in a group with the teacher monitoring all aspects of the child's work. There is less emphasis on the grade achieved and more on actual mastery of the material. The teacher moves to new material only when most or all of the children have learned the concepts being taught. This slower pace can be readily attained since the teacher is aware of each child's strengths and weaknesses and teaches accordingly. Often teachers use the "kindergarten" mode of grading, which consists of giving the work back to the child to correct or remaining uncommitted about an answer's correctness (for example, "almost" or "you're close") long after it is appropriate to do so. As a result, the child may not even understand that being "the best" at a particular task is a worthy goal.

During this period the child begins to act as a separate unit, gaining a sense of acceptance from peers and adults outside of the immediate family. Some degree of social acceptance is easy to attain within the small class. Rejection usually occurs from outside rather than within the group, unless a child enters an established self-contained group mid-year. When a self-contained class is housed in a public school, social rejection might thus occur during activities with normally hearing students, but not within the class itself. Under teacher direction it is less likely that small sub-groups evolve. If they do the special education teacher is likely to disband them to include all in the group.

Junior High School (11–13 years)
If no level of mainstreaming is expected, the kind and quality of academic programming will be different from that of other children in the junior high school. Although similar subject areas will be addressed, it is unlikely that the same level of complexity will be involved. The most noticeable difference from the regular curriculum is the absence of demand to produce analytic essays or research papers; the ability to verbally compare and contrast is often beyond the linguistic capabilities of children who require a self-contained placement.

It is possible for self-contained students to be actively involved in extracurricular activities established for the main school population. Sports, clubs, and fine arts may be avenues for the hearing-impaired child to feel part of the regular school program. Socially, such acceptance becomes critical during the preadolescent and adolescent period. The student may enjoy popularity in the self-contained program but remain unrecognized in the greater population of the school. Since peer acceptance is such a critical factor, the student may need to decide to which group he/she wants to be compared. Hearing-impaired students, like those with normal hearing, will typically select the group in which they experience the greatest success.

During preadolescence children begin to develop their male/female identity. If the hearing-impaired program is small, students may have to seek opposite-sex friends outside of it. The students' ability to conform to the norms of their particular community and school is critical to their acceptance outside of the class. For adolescents, being one of the group is a top priority.

High School (14–18 years)
Academically, the high school student in a self-contained class does not experience the fragmentation intrinsic to the departmentalization of the regular curriculum. Due to the low incidence of hearing loss, even the largest programs have only a few stu-

dents in the upper grades. As a consequence, only one or two teachers are responsible for the entire high school curriculum. To compensate for this difficulty, many districts elect to send their students to large residential high school programs, or decide to mainstream the students with the assistance of an interpreter and/or notetakers.

Since the public schools are responsible for hearing-impaired students until twenty-one years of age (P.L. 94-142), they have an extended period of time to acquire the same skills as normally hearing students. The self-contained high school program, although lacking the variety and depth of the regular classroom, provides a safe, protected haven for learning such skills.

The student is at a disadvantage when mainstreaming is first attempted at the high school level, since he/she will not have had the opportunity to develop the coping strategies demanded by such a competitive environment. On the other hand, it may have taken the student until that point in his/her school career to acquire the necessary skills to fully participate in either a vocational/technical school or an academic high school.

Service Provision

The services described below are generally included as part of the regular program in self-contained classrooms and children are not taken out of class for them. This allows the professional involved to closely coordinate remedial activities with classroom content.

Auditory Learning

Auditory learning is not an issue when students do not routinely wear their amplification and feel they have little need for using their hearing for the most rudimentary purposes. Before auditory training can be effective, students must be convinced that hearing and "listening" are important.

When addressed, auditory learning is often a separate activity incorporated into the curriculum. The teacher has many opportunities to foster auditory growth due to the small number of students in the class. The list below includes suggestions for teachers in self-contained classrooms to stimulate auditory learning within daily interactions and activities. It assumes that the classroom for the hearing impaired is acoustically modified so that optimal listening conditions exist and that the teachers are aware of the changes necessary to communicate with these children.

Provide access to rich auditory-verbal environment.

Provide opportunities for the child to alert to speech through auditory means.

Call attention to and label naturally occurring environmental sounds (telephone, bells, knock).

Call attention to other children's responses and the need to monitor when they are occurring.

Introduce "listening" activities using classroom vocabulary or experience story charts after they have been introduced in combined mode.

Present familiar routines (attendance, job assignments) listen-only when the vocabulary is familiar and highly predictable.

Provide opportunities for student to function without interpreter as he/she demonstrates the ability to receive speech.

Modifications in Expectations

The expectation that auditory behaviors will occur is required if the desired result is to be achieved.

1. Expect child to alert and respond via audition instead of tactile or visual means.

2. Expect child to act when fire drill sounds or bell rings, after "learning" the sound.

3. Expect student to alert to his/her name when called.

4. Expect student to gradually be aware of other students' vocal responses and overtures.

5. Expect child to receive information directly from teacher via listening and lipreading, especially when interpreter is not present.

6. Expect child to rely on speech to answer/ask questions and to make comments.

7. Expect an increase in conversational participation during social interaction.

Parents can also be enlisted in the effort. By expecting and insisting on full-time amplification use at home, they ensure that the child has the raw material on which to build his/her auditory skills.

Speech Remediation

Speech production remediation is accomplished as a separate subject area within the class. Often the classroom teacher determines the deficit areas and plans speech lessons around them. If a speech-language pathologist is available, he/she usually provides individual sessions addressing the suprasegmental and segmental aspects of speech production, and consults with the classroom teacher regarding speech targets, activities, and progress.

The self-contained nature of the class provides many opportunities for the teacher to expect and insist on optimal speech skills from the student. Each word used in social studies, math, reading, science, and language arts can be exploited as a speech target. It is only with vigilance that the speech produced by students in self-contained classes remains intelligible since the overall communicative demand is low. When all the conversational partners have similar "poor speech intelligibility," students resort to a more efficient communication mode to transmit their ideas and wishes (usually gesture, sign, or physical manipulation). Further, if amplification is not used, there can be no self-monitoring of speech production.

Language Learning
Language lessons are included in the curriculum and typically presented and reinforced in a spoken and graphic format. The classroom teacher has many opportunities to reinforce appropriate use of syntax, vocabulary, morphology, and pragmatics within classroom activities. Care should be taken to present the word/form in both written and graphic mode. If the written symbol is always present the student never has to rely on its spoken representation.

Academic Skills
The classroom teacher is responsible for teaching and reinforcing concepts. The class moves on to new topics when the majority of the students have mastered the lesson objectives. Thus primary teaching and tutorial are included in the same class, not conducted separately as in a mainstream placement.

Social Skills
Often hearing-impaired students who are academically grouped together spread inappropriate social behaviors, such as physically getting attention, invading personal space, or negatively commenting on other peoples' attributes. Since the majority of the day students are in the company only of other hearing-impaired students, this continuation of "hearing-impaired" behaviors is not surprising. Increased contact with normally hearing students helps age-appropriate social behaviors to emerge. Social skill development has recently been included in the curriculum of self-contained classes, especially those that propose to eventually place students in mainstream settings. Through role-playing and discussion, the knowledge of appropriate/inappropriate behaviors is enacted.

The teacher needs to find opportunities to integrate the self-contained students into the nonacademic activities of the regular classes. It may be possible to invite the other students for class parties and special celebrations. It is good practice to preview and practice the social skills involved in the party scenario. The other students in the school can be invited to "special days" where the entire day/week focuses on one concept. One school held "100" week where all of the special activities involved the number 100.

Parent Involvement
Parents have to make an extra effort to be involved in the education of children in self-contained classes. Unless a system is established for communication between the school and home, parents will remain uninformed and only peripherally involved. It is especially important that they broaden the student's life experiences and related language through vacations, activities, museum visits, field trips, and entertainment.

AUDITORY MANAGEMENT

Hearing Aid Evaluation (HAE)

All school-age children can give both objective and subjective information that is invaluable in the selection and fitting of amplification. Although older children are capable of directly participating in hearing aid evaluation, the reports of parents and teachers about everyday functioning are critical. For example, the school speech-language pathologist may notice that the child who previously produced a clear /s/ sound has stopped doing so with newly fit hearing aids. The astute audiologist will recognize that this speech production change may reflect a need to change the hearing aid setting.

Communication between clinical and school personnel must take place when selecting and fitting school-worn amplification. If an FM system with an adaptive coupling is to be used, the personal hearing aids must accommodate it. The clinical audiologist cannot be expected to know about school-worn amplification unless informed by parents and school personnel.

By school age, the child with hearing loss and his/her family should be familiar with the need for and use of personal amplification and have a good sense of how to maximize residual hearing. There is also a continuing need to clinically assess the child's hearing status and performance with amplification. Such assessments should be recommended in the child's IEP as a regular component of auditory management. Parents continue throughout the educational process to have questions about use of hearing, goals and expectations with amplification, and the effects of hearing loss. Those questions are best addressed by the school and clinical personnel.

Recommending Classroom Amplification

A major transition may occur during the school years when classroom amplification is recommended for the first time. The advantages of a wireless FM system over traditional hearing aids may be obvious to the speech, language and hearing professionals (see Chapter 2), but the child, parents, and other educational personnel may need to be persuaded of them.

Even when there are no specific objections to or questions about the decision to provide special classroom amplification, a demonstration of the need for an FM system can avert potential problems. Table 7.1 explains the major purpose of an FM system—creating a positive signal-to-noise ratio, regardless of proximity to the sound source—as well as techniques to show that advantage (Ross, Brackett, and Maxon, 1991).

Specific FM Recommendations

Amplification requirements—including frequency response characteristics, output limits, gain requirements, and earmold modifications—are essential to consider when making decisions about the specific make, model, and coupling method of the FM. Although hearing aid electroacoustic characteristics are typically recommended by an audiologist, the same may not be true of FM systems. When such decisions are made by education professionals or the FM manufacturer's representative and not an audiologist, inappropriate fittings result (Maxon, Brackett and van den Berg, 1991).

The child's audiologist should be a direct part of the decision-making process in FM recommendation, selection and fitting. Initially, he/she should decide on the type of FM (traditional or with adaptive coupling) that will work best considering the child's amplification and educational needs. Table 7.2 lists some of the considerations the audiologist must review in making the appropriate recommendations (Maxon, in press).

Validating the FM Fitting

Once an FM is in use it is important to ensure that it is fit correctly and being used properly. The validation has four basic components: clinical assessment, classroom observation, performance assessment, and child report.

Clinical assessment is like the traditional hearing aid fitting, measuring functional gain (aided versus unaided warble tone thresholds) of the environmental microphones and the microphone/transmitter. Receptive speech intelligibility, especially through the remote microphone and in a background of noise, can provide valuable suprathreshold information. Real ear measures show how much sound is actually being delivered to the child's ears across frequencies.

Classroom observation is a critical component and should take place in the various educational settings in which the child functions. An FM system may provide great benefit in the regular classroom setting, but cause problems if kept on at recess or in the cafeteria. The only method of assessing the appropriateness in the different settings is through direct observation. Observations allow for resolution of problems and ensure better classroom performance because immediate feedback can be given to the teachers about their microphone technique.

The performance assessment that was presented in Table 7.1 (items 1-3) should be carried out as part of the child's annual review, including receptive speech intelligibility and comprehension of connected discourse in difficult listening conditions. The child should be encouraged to report problems either directly to the classroom teacher, or to his/her case manager. With open communication, problematic situations will not be allowed to build over time.

All individuals involved in FM use should be aware of how it functions best. They should also know the situations that interfere with its benefits. The point of an FM system is to improve the signal-to-noise ratio (S/N), but not at the expense of the child's access to all environmental sound. The environmental microphones are the child's only access to his/her own voice, other children's voices, and environmental sounds. There are therefore very few times that the environmental microphones should be deactivated. Unfortunately it is a common misconception that if a good

Table 7.1   The advantages of an FM system and methods of demonstration (Adapted from Maxon in press; Ross, Brackett, and Maxon, 1991).

1. **Advantage:** An improvement in receptive speech intelligibility or paragraph comprehension over hearing aids at a *distance* from the sound source.

   Demonstration: Compare receptive speech discrimination scores (auditory only). Present monosyllabic words (e.g., Boothroyd's isophonemic lists) in a normal conversational voice with child standing ten feet from the speaker. Obtain a percent correct score using hearing aids and a percent correct score using the FM system with the remote microphone/transmitter.

   Use a commercially available video or audiotape that demonstrates the advantage.

2. **Advantage:** An improvement in receptive speech intelligibility or paragraph comprehension over hearing aids in a background of *noise.*

   Demonstration: Compare receptive speech discrimination scores (auditory only). Present monosyllabic words (e.g., Boothroyd's isophonemic lists) in a normal conversational voice with child standing three feet from the speaker with noise in the background. Obtain a percent correct score using hearing aids and a percent correct score using the FM system with the remote microphone/transmitter.

   Use a commercially available video or audiotape that demonstrates the advantage.

3. **Advantage:** An improvement in receptive speech intelligibility or paragraph comprehension over hearing aids when listening at a *distance* from the sound source *and* when in a background of *noise.*

   Demonstration: Compare receptive speech discrimination scores (auditory only). Present monosyllabic words (e.g., Boothroyd's isophonemic lists) in a normal conversational voice with child standing ten feet from the speaker with noise in the background. Obtain a percent correct score using hearing aids and a percent correct score using the FM system with the remote microphone/transmitter.

   Use a commercially available video or audiotape that demonstrates the advantage.

4. **Advantage:** Child's classroom performance/interaction over using hearing aids.

   Demonstration: Teacher's report before and during FM use. Child's report before and during FM use. Case manager's observations before and during FM use.

Table 7.2 Some issues audiologists should consider when recommending specific makes and models of FM systems (Maxon in press).

FM Type	Considerations
Traditional Unit	1. Child's unit is sturdy.
	2. Controls are accessible.
	3. Easy to troubleshoot.
	4. Easy to maintain.
	5. Easy adjustment of electroacoustic characteristics.
	6. Environmental signal is received at chest level.
	7. Cords are a vulnerable component.
Traditional Unit with Ear-level Mikes	1. Environmental signal is received at ear level.
	2. Other qualities of a traditional unit are maintained.
Neck Loop Coupling	1. Environmental signal may be received at ear level.
	2. No direct connection between child's unit and hearing aids.
	3. Hearing aids must have a good quality telecoil.
	4. An environmental microphone is needed if no M/T switch on hearing aids.
	5. Output, gain, and frequency response of hearing aid's telecoil may be altered by the coupling (see Chapter 2).
	6. FM-to-environmental microphone ratio may be altered by the coupling.
	7. Troubleshooting is difficult. Must maintain hearing aid close to neck loop (see Appendix).
	8. Hearing aid breakdown affects classroom amplification.
Direct Audio Input	1. Environmental signal is received at ear level.
	2. Hearing aids must allow for this coupling of boot/shoe, or direct cord input.
	3. Boot/shoe must be appropriate for FM unit and hearing aids (see Chapter 2).
	4. Connecting cord must be appropriate for hearing aid and boot/shoe (see Chapter 2).
	5. Output, gain, and frequency response of hearing aids may be altered by the coupling (see Chapter 2).
	6. FM-to-environmental microphone ratio may be altered by the coupling.
	7. Troubleshooting is difficult. Two people are necessary to determine if FM transmitter is functioning (see Appendix).
	8. Hearing aid breakdown affects classroom amplification.

signal-to-noise ratio is provided when the environmental microphones are working, that an even better one will be attained without them and this will be better for the child.

The microphone/transmitter should always be functioning when the speaker is directing his/her voice to the child, but should be deactivated when the child is not meant to hear what is being said. Thus the microphone/transmitter should be used by the speaker in the following situations: (1) the teacher is the primary sound source for the child; (2) the teacher repeats what the child says; (3) the teacher passes it to other speakers; (4) another child is giving an oral report or "show and tell"; (5) there is an assembly speaker; or (6) there is a tour guide on a class trip. Conversely, the transmitter should be deactivated when the teacher is directing his/her voice to someone other than the child with hearing loss. Some examples include when the teacher is talking to another adult or child, is engaged in a nonteaching activity, or is talking to a group of children exclusive of the FM user.

The FM system can also be used to couple an electronic audio source via the auxiliary input of the microphone/transmitter. In this way the child can gain access to the audio track of a televised program, including videotapes, or one presented on an audiotape recorder.

Troubleshooting

Daily troubleshooting of the child's amplification, both personal and classroom-type, should be routinely incorporated into his/her IEP. The information in the Appendix should be adapted to the amplification of each child. To facilitate the troubleshooting procedures, careful documentation about the child's amplification should be kept on file, either with the person designated to conduct the troubleshooting program or with the child's case manager. Such files should include the tone, output, amplification, volume settings, and earmold design for both personal hearing aids and the FM system. Directions for charging and use of the FM system should also be readily available.

Use of Residual Hearing

The use of amplification assumes that the child will make maximal use of available residual hearing. Auditory management should be included in the IEP (see Chapter 4) regardless of the child's communication mode or educational setting. For older children, emphasis should be placed on the use of hearing for speech reception and perception. Specific suggestions for designing an auditory training program based on reception of the acoustic cues of speech are presented in Chapter 4. A carefully planned program should be developed based on the individual child's skills and the communicative demands of the classroom and daily living environment.

SUMMARY

There needs to be a logical progression from evaluation to management as the student's strengths and weaknesses are delineated and addressed. A placement should be selected that challenges the student educationally yet has the services required to support his/her efforts. Also, frequent reassessments are necessary to evaluate the effectiveness of the placement and to recommend changes in placement or services when appropriate. Movement to a less restrictive or more protective environment should be considered when a student evidences the need. Effective preparation for dealing with the communicative and knowledge requirements of the world is the basis on which an educational program should be developed.

References

Brackett, D. & Maxon, A.B. (1986). Service delivery alternatives for the mainstreamed hearing-impaired child. *Language, Speech, and Hearing Services in the Schools* 17, 115-25.

Davis, J. & Hardick, E. (1981). *Rehabilitative Audiology for Children and Adults* (p. 330). New York, NY: John Wiley & Sons.

Erber, N.P. (1982). *Auditory Training.* Washington, DC: A.G. Bell Association.

Maxon, A.B. (in press) Selection and use of FM systems for school-age children. In M. Ross (Ed.) *FM Auditory Training Systems,* Parkton, MD: York Press

Maxon, A.B. & Brackett, D. (1987). The hearing-impaired child in regular schools. *Seminars in Speech and Language,* 8, 393-413.

Maxon, A.B. & Brackett, D. (1991). FM use for children with mild hearing loss: Necessity or luxury. *Proceedings of 6th International SHHH Convention,* 53-56.

Maxon, A.B., Brackett, D. & van den Berg, S.A. (1991). Classroom amplification use: A national long-term study. *Language, Speech and Hearing Services in the Schools,* 22,4,242-253.

Northcott, W.H. (1973). *The Hearing Impaired Child in the Regular Classroom: Preschool, Primary, and Secondary Years.* Washington, DC: A.G. Bell Association.

Paul, P.V. & Quigley, S.P. (1990). *Education and Deafness.* White Plains, NY: Longman Publishers.

Ross, M., Brackett, D. & Maxon, A.B. (1991). *Assessment and Management of Hearing-Impaired Children: Principles and Practices.* Austin, TX: Pro-Ed.

8

Psychosocial, Familial, and Cultural Issues

INTRODUCTION

The benefits of careful planning for communication, auditory, and educational management may be compromised when a hearing-impaired child does not have a positive self-image or a circle of friends. Further, a family's cultural, social, and financial status must be an integral part of programming to avoid any related problems. Although interference from family, social, and community factors may be potentially greater for mainstreamed children, they may also exist for children in self-contained placements.

THE HEARING-IMPAIRED CHILD

Due to the ease of data collection, most of the literature pertaining to the socio-emotional development of hearing-impaired children is restricted to those who are in residential and day programs. Few studies explore the socialization of mainstreamed hearing-impaired children. Such children have communicative and academic skills that span a wide range (Brackett and Maxon, 1986; Davis, Shepard, Stelmachowicz and Gorga, 1981; Maxon and Brackett, 1981); and, it can thus be anticipated that their social skills will also be quite disparate, requiring careful individual planning.

Infants and Toddlers

Although their scope of socialization tends to be limited, some daily living factors are likely to affect developing children and impact on their future socialization. Communication and the demands for interaction are major issues within the family. The type of communication base parents establish with their child is dependent on their interaction style. During this early interactive period parents and children influence each other's emotional behaviors (Parke and Asher, 1983). Even children with very limited communication can thus affect the parent/child interactive pattern. For example, parental input tends to decrease when an infant is nonresponsive.

Decreased parental input reduces the linguistic stimulation crucial for language acquisition. Further, mothers of children with lower-level linguistic skills tend to be more directive than those whose children are better communicators (White and White, 1984). Limited pragmatic and social skills, which impact on later socialization patterns, are the outcome of reduced parental input in the early years.

Preschool Children

Young children with severe to profound hearing losses often have delayed social skills due to prolonged dependence and low self-confidence. Further, such children have difficulty developing an internal locus of control, experience social delays and isolation, and have more behavioral adjustment problems than peers with normal hearing. Parental expectations may be responsible for some of these differences because parents tend to make fewer demands and intervene more when their child experiences frustration. Such interaction limits feelings of success that derive from the child's employing his/her own coping skills (Heller, 1991). Thus dependence on parents and familiar adults is fostered, immature behaviors prolonged, and parental protectiveness reinforced. The cycle develops and is difficult to break, especially since younger children are unaware that their behavior is different from what is expected.

When parents are aware of the long-term negative effects of early dependence, they can work to change it. For example, they can assign age-appropriate chores for the child to do around the house. Success in completing tasks independently in the protectiveness of the home can be rewarding for both child and parents. It will be easier for parents to give their child responsibilities when they do not feel pity for the child, but realistically accept his/her strengths and weaknesses.

Aside from effecting interaction with parents, hearing status may also have an effect on a child's position in social groups (Arnold and Tremblay, 1979). For example, problems may arise in integrated educational settings if normally hearing children choose to avoid the hearing-impaired child. Language compatibility has a greater influence on interaction than the presence of hearing loss (Brackett and Henniges, 1976). The child with age-appropriate (or at least group-appropriate) language skills can become well integrated into social groups. Thus, the interaction of communication abilities and socialization that is established in infancy continues to have an impact throughout the life of an individual with hearing loss.

School-age Children

Once children enter school on a full-time basis they are routinely forced to interact with different people in a variety of settings. A summary of the interactions particular to mainstreamed children are presented in Table 8.1 (Maxon, Brackett, and van den Berg, 1991). It can be seen that most of the problem areas are related to the child's being "different" from the other children. Those differences (wearing ampli-

Table 8.1   Mainstream situations that are a potential source of social difficulties for the child with hearing loss. Adapted from the work of Maxon, Brackett, and van den Berg (1991).

Situation	Potential Problem
Single child with hearing loss in school.	No older hearing-impaired children with whom to identify.
	No hearing-impaired children with whom to share experiences.
	Normally hearing children are unfamiliar with hearing loss.
Use of classroom amplification.	Singles the child out as different.
	Source of derision.
	If used incorrectly, can interfere with communication in social situations.
Being taken out of class for support services.	Singles child out as different.
	May miss social opportunities.
Communication breakdown in academic and social situations.	Source of derision.
	Normally hearing child may stop trying.
	Hearing-impaired child may stop trying.
Difficult listening conditions.	May lead to communication breakdown.
	May cause child to remove self from groups.

fication, receiving speech and language services, having communication problems) are resolvable and must be addressed through a management program.

A management program that includes coping strategies for the child can help tremendously. However, the goal is not to make hearing-impaired children view themselves as normally hearing, but to make them cognizant of the attributes that define them as valued individuals. Socialization will take a more natural course when they accept how hearing impairment makes them different, while realizing that it is not their only descriptive characteristic.

The demands and opportunities for social interaction must also be considered for the child placed in a self-contained class. Typically, there are limited contacts with normally hearing peers and older students to serve as models for social interaction. The situations presented in Table 8.2 differ from those applicable to the mainstreamed child, primarily because the child in the self-contained class is automatically a part of an established group. Most problems are associated with interaction outside of the confines and comforts of the classroom.

Regardless of their educational placement, school-age hearing-impaired children seem to be aware of their social difficulties. They report feeling like outsiders

Table 8.2 Self-contained situations that are a potential source of social problems for the child with hearing loss.

Situation	Potential Problem
One of many children with hearing loss in the school.	No contact with peers with good speech and language. No need to make an effort to establish traditional social skills.
Being educated in a protected environment.	No contact with peers who are unlike themselves. No contact with adults who are not understanding of their problems. No preparation for the "hearing world."

and requiring a teacher to mediate their classroom interactions, especially with normally hearing peers (Kennedy, Northcott, McCauley, and Williams, 1978). School-age hearing-impaired children differ from their normally hearing peers in that they (1) are shy, withdrawn, poorly motivated, and dependent (McCrane, 1980); (2) act like aggressive or uncooperative normally hearing children (McCrane, 1980); (3) lack social/emotional maturity, self-confidence, and initiative (Meadow, 1980); (4) have difficulty in peer relationships with a strong desire to please others; and (5) have exaggerated physical aggression (Meadow, 1980).

Like those of preschoolers, the communicative patterns of school-age children impact on their social interactions. Younger (first through sixth grade) partially mainstreamed children tend to interact more with teachers than with peers (Anita, 1982). This continuation of adult dependence is perceived as negative by normally hearing peers. By spending more time with adults, the hearing-impaired child limits his/her opportunities for peer-to-peer communication.

Decreased social contacts affect the way hearing-impaired children perceive their social skills and status. Older mainstreamed children (eight to fifteen years) describe themselves as less popular and unlikely to be selected as friend of normally hearing peers (Loeb and Sargiani, 1986). All of these perceived and actual socialization problems may have their roots in deficient language systems. Their lower language levels may cause such children to be perceived as younger children with normal hearing (Maxon, Brackett and van den Berg, 1991). For example, hearing-impaired adolescent girls express their annoyance or frustration by physically acting out their behavior, in contrast to normally hearing teenagers who verbally mediate any argument. There are fewer opportunities to develop social relationships that rely on interactive skills for school-age hearing-impaired children who have reduced linguistic ability than there are for normally hearing children. Without the opportunity to employ and refine their social abilities, the social development of such children is delayed (Fitz-Gerald and Reeves Fitz-Gerald, 1987).

Adolescent hearing-impaired children experience greater conflict than normally hearing peers particularly in their interactions with parents. It is not surprising that parents who discouraged independence in early childhood are later unwilling to allow their children the freedom to advance without assistance through the standard teenage rites of passage. Adolescents in that situation want such freedom yet have not had the opportunity to develop the skills necessary to attain it. They find themselves overly resentful of parental restraints, yet unable to break away.

The typical complaint of adolescents that parents do not understand the problems and pressures they experience, may be exacerbated when hearing-impaired children have normally hearing parents. In that instance, teenagers already frustrated and angry over parental limitations feel the additional burden of having parents who have never coped with hearing impairment on a daily basis (Cohen, 1978). When they say, "You don't know how I feel," they are correct on several counts.

All teenagers rebel against parents, families, and the morals of their culture/community. A common act of defiance is to adopt overt mannerisms, dress codes, and beliefs that are contrary to those of their parents. When the child is the only hearing-impaired family member, he/she may manifest such rebellion by shunning the communication modality "approved" and chosen by the parents in favor of a different one, used in a challenging manner. A teenager who has always been mainstreamed and never had hearing-impaired friends may express a strong desire to become involved with clubs for the hearing impaired, or show a particular interest in "deaf culture" issues.

The clashes that develop in adolescence should not be overly exaggerated. Parents may be able to relieve some of the pressure as the child matures by relinquishing their stronghold. Although the child's changes may make the parents and family very uncomfortable, they must be viewed for what they are—a normal part of the maturational process.

Sexuality

Communicating about sexuality is awkward for both children and parents. Parental concern about discussing sexual issues may be exacerbated when the adolescent or teenager is hearing impaired. Parents have particular difficulty discussing sexual issues when they are: (1) embarrassed or uncomfortable; (2) confused or uninformed; (3) unsure of their own values or feelings; (4) fear that discussion will lead to "trying;" (5) unable to use the child's communication modality to clearly express themselves; and (6) unsure of when or how to begin. They also have difficulty when their child does not ask questions and says he/she knows about sex (Fitz-Gerald and Reeves Fitz-Gerald, 1987).

Questions about sexual and emotional issues are part of a normal developmental process. Whereas younger children ask more factual, biological or mechanical questions, the concerns of older children are relationships, feelings, and dealing with specific situations. Although hearing-impaired children follow normal patterns, they progress at a slightly delayed rate. The delay may be related to language and a difficulty understanding concepts that are typically acquired via the linguistic environment (Fitz-Gerald and Reeves Fitz-Gerald, 1987). Their language delays interfere with learning social behaviors, including those related to sexuality.

School-age children acquire most of their information about sex from peers (Thornburg, 1981), with most normally hearing adolescents gaining more than half their knowledge between the years of twelve and thirteen. At an age when social acceptance is so critical, having a shared level of basic knowledge is imperative. Familiarity with the group-accepted terms for body parts and sexual activity is held in high regard by young teenagers. Hearing loss interferes with learning language incidentally, the way in which most of the "street terms" for sexually-related vocabulary is acquired. Managing this language-based problem is difficult—it is the rare parent or professional who can comfortably familiarize a child with the latest slang related to sexuality.

PARENTS

The hearing-impaired child is, above all, an integral part of a family unit. All families have functions and those functions define the roles of individual members. Parental roles may include those of teacher, health care provider, caretaker, disciplinarian, and material needs provider (Bailey and Simeonsson, 1988). The way in which those roles are shared by the two parents or accepted by the single parent depends on the daily living conditions of the family members. Children have different familial roles that are often determined by age, birth order, gender, number of siblings, and socialization within and outside of the family (Bailey and Simeonsson, 1988).

When a hearing-impaired child is part of a family, parental and sibling roles are dramatically affected by his/her needs. Parents find addressing the needs of the hearing-impaired child so demanding and their training responsibilities so stressful that they can accommodate the other children only with difficulty. Acceptance of a hearing-impaired child into the family unit changes with time. Typically when these children are younger they are easily integrated into the family because their "differences" are less noticeable. When the gap between the child's physical size and language competence unavoidably becomes obvious, family members may feel embarrassment about the child's deficits. The initial stress on the family increases as the individual members are forced to acknowledge that the hearing-impaired child is different and will always be so.

Life changes dramatically for the parents when their child is diagnosed with a hearing loss. Luterman (1979) carefully defines the stages of grieving that parents experience when they learn that the "normal" child no longer exists. They may initially blame the problem on the professional who makes the diagnosis. Although this anger is misdirected, it and the stages of acceptance that follow are healthy. They allow parents and siblings to acknowledge the different path their lives must take to accommodate the hearing-impaired child, and thus help the family to move in a positive direction.

Prior to taking positive action parents may have difficulty accepting help from professionals, family, and friends. They may find comfort in isolating themselves from others because it is easier than coping with all of the demands placed on them. Even explaining the hearing loss, the amplification, and the intricacies of the management program can be overwhelming in the early stages of grieving. Further, parents may turn their attention away from others because they are jealous of any time spent away from their child. Although a "special" parent/child relationship may develop, it may have some negative effects in the long term.

Parents go through this process at the initial diagnosis and every time there is a change in the child's status. However, although the grieving reaction may begin anew, its strength will be less severe during the transition periods outlined in Table 8.3. Parents have a very difficult job. They must establish strong bonds with their child, be demanding yet avoid frustration, provide intense intervention and reinforcement, yet be willing to "let go" when it is appropriate for the child to explore on his/her own. Parents must provide opportunities for their child to develop and practice independent coping skills. By allowing their child to demonstrate this competence, parents empower him/her.

Over the last decade there has been an increase in the number of dual-career and single-parent families. This change from the traditional framework for child-rearing is an additional source of familial stress. In nontraditional families the need for child care services is critical, yet there are few facilities or professionals prepared to deal with hearing-impaired children (Somers, 1987). Even after the child reaches school age, the need to attend to the various evaluations, management services, and meetings can negatively affect a parent's ability to maintain full-time employment.

Table 8.3   Life transitions that may trigger a grieving reaction on the part of parents of children with hearing loss.

Change in hearing status
Change in amplification
Change in educational placement
Change in communication modality
Starting school
Adolescence
Starting work
Acquiring driver's license
Dating

In single-parent families the extra responsibilities associated with the hearing loss are shouldered by only one parent. Further, this individual may be caught between trying to establish personal and professional independence and meeting all of the needs of the hearing-impaired child (Somers, 1987). The single parent experiences greater stress than if there were a spouse or significant other present to share the financial and emotional burdens, as well as the joys.

Culturally Diverse Families

In today's society individuals from minority cultures are expected to have the linguistic and social competence to function in two different worlds. Over one-third of school-age hearing-impaired children are from minority cultures (Center for Assessment and Demographic Studies, 1985-86); how their families cope with hearing loss and immersion into both the majority and minority cultures must be an integral component of their management programs.

The diversity of cultural attitudes about handicapping conditions requires that professionals have a cross-cultural understanding of hearing loss and its effects. For example, some cultural groups regard hearing loss as a medically related issue, while others consider it from a religious perspective. The manner in which parents pursue identification or management differs greatly across the two groups. Therefore, professionals must first understand that families will seek identification, assessment, and management services in accordance with the views of their cultural group (Randall-David, 1989).

The family's willingness to adhere to the proposed management plan once the hearing loss is identified is also culturally bound. In turn, the manner in which the professional interacts with a family is governed by his/her culture, its difference from that of the family, and his/her training in establishing good lines of communication. A commonly cited cultural difference is the perception of time. Whereas in some ethnic groups punctuality is highly valued, in others being at a particular place at the time specified is not viewed as mandatory. Further, time commitments may be prioritized according to differing factors (Randall-David, 1989). For example, a family may have a clinical appointment for a child at 10 a.m. on Monday. On Sunday evening the child's grandmother becomes ill requiring that the mother attend to her. Since reverence for the elder generation takes priority over the needs of younger family members, the mother goes to the grandmother and does not keep the child's appointment.

Although valuing children is a cross-cultural phenomenon, its manifestations differ considerably. Accordingly, families that accept a child's handicapping condition without question and feel little need to affect change may be less enthusiastic about an intervention program than those who have a desire to make their child reach full potential in spite of problems. Professionals can avoid becoming annoyed or angry when confronted with broken appointments or lax application of programming techniques by understanding their cultural derivation.

The roles that family members play are defined and limited by their cultures. For example, the head of the household may be the father, the eldest male, or the mother depending on the ethnic or racial group. Further, the head-of-household's specific functions may range from material needs provider to decision maker, or those functions may be shared. Of particular importance are gender-determined limitations because of the potential communication barriers they create between families and professionals. For example, in some groups females do not engage directly in decision making, remaining instead in the background. In others, all family needs are addressed by the female except earning wages (Randall-David, 1989). The professional must know which parent will take responsibility for acquiring knowledge, scheduling appointments, communicating with school personnel, and implementing home management techniques.

The way in which families view professionals impacts dramatically on the effectiveness of the management program. For example, when females are not expected to be actively involved in decision making, a strong female case manager will have a difficult time working with both male and female family members. Their suggestions may not be accepted, or even given any consideration. Such issues may be compounded when a professional ignores the etiquette peculiar to a particular community. Since some groups require formality in professional situations, any informality of dress or manner is viewed as inappropriate and detracts from the professional's credibility. Further, the professional who attempts to "break accepted codes" will not be successful. For example, obtaining complete case history information can be quite difficult when individuals are reluctant to reveal personal and/ or family information. Pushing for answers to questions will serve to establish a barrier, not rapport.

Professionals must also have strategies for dealing with families of diverse socioeconomic status. The number of low-income families has risen over the last decade, especially those headed by a single parent. Almost half the low-income families in the United States have a woman as head-of-household. When such families include hearing-impaired children they face unique barriers to accessing professional services. Some of those impediments are need for affordable child care, transportation to appointments, communication differences, and feelings of inferiority around professionals (Somers, 1987). Low-income families' problems are exacerbated by an increased disease rate and reduced access to medical care, increasing their need for services they cannot obtain.

SIBLINGS

Siblings of children with hearing loss are an often-overlooked group. A child's established role in the family as well as his/her relationship with the parents changes when a new sibling enters the unit. Further, those roles may change again when the "new" child is diagnosed as medically or physically impaired.

With the identification of hearing impairment parents are forced to change the quality and quantity of interaction with the hearing-impaired child. As they become more "teacher" to that child their relationships with their other children change (Atkins, 1987). Because of the time demands as well as associated stress, the increased focus on the needs of the child with hearing loss reduces the attention parents can give to their normally hearing child(ren). They simply do not have as much time and energy to cope with the problems of their normally hearing children after coping with those of the hearing-impaired child. Siblings face this decreased attention on a daily basis. For example, they see that the majority of family discussions center on the child with hearing loss and that their needs are secondary. Although such perceptions may in some cases be exaggerated, they are not inaccurate. As parents address the needs of the hearing-impaired child they tend to excuse behaviors that they would not accept in their normally hearing children. Further, parents tend to be more lenient and protective of the child with hearing loss, while continuing to make strict demands on the normally hearing children.

Some siblings may be faced with shouldering an unfair burden to achieve in areas unattainable by the hearing-impaired child. Or the child may burden him/herself in an effort to compensate for the parents' disappointment in the limitations of the hearing-impaired child. Siblings may be assigned responsibilities as part of the programming, such as monitoring homework or making an experience book. When this happens, the sibling can harbor resentment, particularly when the success of the hearing-impaired child is noticed without recognition of the sibling's contribution.

Even when a sibling is eager to work with a brother or sister with hearing loss, the relationship that ensues can be one of dependency as the normally hearing partner becomes "caretaker." The sibling may then be expected to take the hearing-impaired child along on social occasions and to make explanations about the hearing impairment. Such social situations are another burden for siblings who find questions about their sibling uncomfortable to handle (Atkins, 1987).

ADDRESSING SPECIFIC NEEDS

Support Groups

Group meetings are effective for encouraging discussion of common concerns and sharing strategies for coping with common problems.

Hearing-impaired children, particularly those in mainstream settings, have a need to understand their similarity with others. Although skills and specific problems can vary widely across individuals, there are commonalities of experience. For example, acknowledging the problems associated with using amplification in noisy environments helps a child recognize that he/she is not peculiar—it is not the child's skills or amplification that is at fault, but the environment. Other children can provide strategies for coping with noise that cannot be reduced.

An opportunity to interact with older children and adults with hearing loss shows the child that "life goes on" and that a variety of educational and vocational options are available. Coping strategies proffered by an individual who has lived through similar problems and has survived are more likely to be adopted than if they were presented by a normally hearing parent or teacher.

Although sibling groups are uncommon, they are effective. Too often siblings have no outlet for sharing the guilt associated with being "healthy" and wishing their hearing-impaired sibling would disappear. When establishing parent or child groups professionals should also include one for siblings. Even if meetings occur only semi-annually, they provide an opportunity to express frustration, embarrassment, and concern about hearing-impaired siblings.

Parent groups help families separate problems associated with hearing loss from those that can be attributed to age and gender. Too often all problems are blamed on the hearing loss without consideration given to the child's developmental level. It is particularly important that parents understand that a child's basic personality is not easily changed, nor should it be. A shy child cannot be made outgoing and should not be forced into social situations that are uncomfortable. In this instance it is not the child's language that affects socialization, but inherent reticence about interacting with peers or adults. Providing information about legal options and advocacy is a particularly important support mechanism. Specific information for parents is presented in Chapter 10.

Children in Transition

The teenager with hearing loss is faced with dating, sexuality, maturation into adulthood, and deciding on vocational or continued educational options. All of these "real life" issues are affected by communicative competence and must be handled accordingly. The child with better skills and greater social maturity will move more easily into the adult-like aspects of life. The expectations that have been realized throughout the child's life evolve into life decisions during such periods of transition.

Group discussions and sharing of information can be particularly helpful during transition periods. Even the mundane problems of amplification can be handled effectively by group meetings. For example, using an FM system can be resisted in junior high school even when it was accepted readily in elementary school. Openly confronting FM-related problems, talking about the embarrassment of feeling different, yet acknowledging the auditory need for classroom amplification become the basis for developing strategies related to the cosmetic issues.

Graduation from high school is a major transition for all children. Those who are moving into vocational training can benefit from interaction with working adults.

The hearing-impaired adults can explain the importance of being prepared not only with vocational/professional skills but also in communicating with the employer and co-workers. Further, they can focus the high school student on appropriate vocational goals while not erecting artificial boundaries to career options. Often parents and professionals severely limit a student's choices because they want to protect him/her from rejection. Surely not every vocation is open to a hearing-impaired child due to auditory demands, but the career opportunities that are excluded from consideration should be only those that the child cannot manage. The individual's strengths and weaknesses should be the basis of vocational guidance, not the hearing loss itself.

Some mainstreamed children decide after graduation from regular education high school that they will benefit from a college program that has support services for the hearing impaired. They may do so because of a perception that other types of higher education do not afford a student special services. All students should be cognizant of the various options available and how to access services in "mainstreamed" higher education settings. Considering the educational and academic demands of different universities is as important as it was for earlier schooling options. The benefits and drawbacks of the various settings should be carefully explored before a final choice is made.

Child Abuse

Children with handicapping conditions are considered particularly vulnerable to child abuse (Krents, Schulman and Brenner, 1987), in part because families in which stress levels are high exhibit a greater incidence of child abuse (Straus, 1980). Parents of hearing-impaired children certainly suffer from stressful living conditions. The long-term, irreversible nature of hearing loss can cause parents to feel overwhelmed and perhaps hopeless at times. Such daily living situations have the potential of increasing the incidence of abuse in families with hearing-impaired children.

Due to their language deficits, hearing-impaired children may have difficulty understanding what is taking place in either heterosexual or homosexual encounters. They are unable to understand innuendo, and may unwittingly display provocative behavior. Further, their immaturity and dependence make them eager to please others, particularly adults. All of these situations make the hearing-impaired child a more likely target for sexual abuse.

There have been efforts to establish programs to make children knowledgeable about sexual and physical abuse. However, few if any of these programs are directed to children with hearing loss. Their communication problems make it more difficult for them to fully express their concerns about these situations and to understand their ability to help prevent them. If groups or programs are established to help children with hearing loss, they must consider their communication needs.

SUMMARY

In the final analysis it is important to remember Stoker's (1991) explanation that the range of personality differences in people with hearing loss is like that for people with normal hearing. "The biological difference between hearing-impaired and normally-hearing people is so slight, that the logical destiny for all should be as members of the general diversity of the human race, not as separate autonomous cultures forever separated." (p.6). Efforts in management should address the between-group similarities as well as the differences.

References

Anita, S.D. (1982). Social interaction of partially mainstreamed hearing-inmpaired children. *American Annals of the Deaf* 127, 18-25.

Arnold, D. & Tremblay, A. (1979). Interaction of deaf and hearing preschooler children. *Journal of Communication Disorders.* 12, 245-251.

Atkins, D.V. (1987). Siblings of the hearing impaired: Perspectives for parents. *Families and Their Hearing-Impaired Children. The Volta Review* 89:5, 32-45.

Bailey, D.B. & Simeonsson, R.J. (1988). *Family Assessment in Early Intervention.* Columbus, OH: Merrill Publishing Company.

Brackett, D. & Henniges, M. (1976). Communicative interaction of preschool hearing-impaired children in an integrated setting. *Volta Review* 78, 276-285.

Brackett, D. & Maxon, A.B. (1986). Service delivery alternatives for the mainstreamed hearing-impaired child. *Language, Speech, and Hearing Services in the Schools* 17, 115-25.

Center for Assessment and Demographic Studies (1985-86). The Annual Survey of Hearing-Impaired Children and Youth, 1985-86 School Year (unpublished report). Washington, DC: Gallaudet University.

Cohen, O.P. (1978). The deaf adolescent: Who am I? *The Volta Review* 80, 265-274.

Davis, J.M., Shepard, N.T., Stelmachowicz, P.G. & Gorga, M.P. (1981). Characteristics of hearing-impaired children in the public schools: Part I, Demographic data. *Journal of Speech and Hearing Disorders* 46:2, 123-129.

Fitz-Gerald, M. & Reeves Fitz-Gerald, D. (1987). Parents' involvement in the sex education of their children. *Families and Their Hearing-Impaired Children, The Volta Review* 89, 96-110.

Heller, P.J. (1991). Yes I can! Building self-esteem and self-reliance for hearing impaired preschoolers. Presented at SHHH Convention, Denver CO.

Kennedy, P., Northcott, W., McCauley, R. & Williams, S.N. (1978). Longitudinal sociometric and cross-sectional data on mainstreaming hearing-impaired children. *Volta Review* 78, 71-82.

Krents, E., Shulman, V. & Brenner, S. (1987). Child abuse and the disabled child: Perspectives for parents. *Families and Their Hearing-Impaired Children. The Volta Review* 89,78-91.

Loeb, R., & Sargiani, P. (1986). The impact of hearing impairment on self-perception of children. *The Volta Review,* 1,89-99.

Luterman, D. (1979). *Counseling Parents of Hearing-Impaired Children.* Boston, MA: Little, Brown and Company.

Maxon, A.B. & Brackett, D. (1981). Inservice training for public school speech-language pathologists. In I. Hochberg, H. Levitt & M.J. Osberger (Eds.) *Speech for the Hearing-Impaired: Research, Training and Personnel Preparation.* Baltimore, MD: University Park Press.

Maxon, A.B., Brackett, D. & van den Berg, S.A. (1991). Self-perception of socialization: The effects of hearing status, age, and gender. *Volta Review* 93:1, 15-17.

McCane, N.P. (1980). Responding to classroom behavior problems among deaf children. *American Annals of the Deaf* 125, 902-905.

Meadow, K.P. (1980). *Deafness and Child Development.* Berkeley, CA: University of California Press.

Parke, R.D., & Asher, S.R. (1983). Social and personality development. *Annual Review of Psychology* 34, 465-509.

Randall-David, E. (1989). *Strategies for Working with Culturally Diverse Communities and Clients.* Bethesda, MD: The Association for the Care of Children's Health.

Somers, M.N. (1987). Parenting in the 1980s: Programming perspectives and issues. *Families and Their Hearing-Impaired Children. The Volta Review* 89, 68-77

Stoker, R.G. (1991). Self awareness and the role of hearing-impaired people. *Volta Review* 93:1, 5-6.

Straus, M.A. (1980). Stress and physical child abuse. *Child Abuse and Neglect.* 4, 75-88.

Thornburg, H.D. (1981). Adolescent sources of information on sex. *Journal of School Health,* 274-277.

White, S.J. & White, R.E.C. (1984). The deaf imperative: Characteristics of maternal input to hearing-impaired children. *Topics in Language Disorders.* 4, 38-49.

9

Children with Conductive, Mild, and Unilateral Hearing Loss

INTRODUCTION

Hearing impairment in children is commonly defined as permanent, bilateral, sensorineural hearing loss of significant degree (greater than 40dB HL). Children with conductive, unilateral, or milder degrees of hearing loss are typically given less attention in the literature. This is pardoxical considering that the latter group exists in much greater numbers. Due to the lack of available research, professionals working with hearing-impaired infants, toddlers, and school-age children may be unaware of the need to intervene early with this population.

Over the last decade it has been demonstrated that children with: (1) fluctuating hearing loss related to middle ear disease; (2) hearing levels between 20dB and 40dB HL (either conductive or sensorineural); and (3) unilateral hearing loss will exhibit long-term negative effects from their hearing impairments. The underlying issue for all three groups is that in order to develop good language and speech perception skills, a child must receive a consistent, clear speech signal. Further, to develop good auditory perceptual skills, particularly binaural, the signal must be relatively equal in both ears. Therefore, the residual effects of these hearing losses may be manifest in children in any one of the three groups as they reach the demanding educational environment of elementary school.

CHILDREN WITH CONDUCTIVE HEARING LOSS, SPECIFICALLY THOSE WITH RECURRENT OR CHRONIC MIDDLE EAR DISEASE RESULTING IN LONG-TERM OR FLUCTUATING HEARING LOSS.

Incidence

Children with chronic or recurrent fluctuating conductive hearing loss related to middle ear disease and effusion are at risk for communication and academic problems. Otitis media (middle ear disease) is the most common disease of early child-

Table 9.1 Children who are at greater risk for acquiring middle ear disease than those in the general population.

AGE: Children under the age of seven, with peak occurrence between zero and twenty-four months.

PHYSICAL CONDITIONS: Children with craniofacial anomalies, including clefts of the palate.

SYNDROMES: Children with Down Syndrome or syndromes related to anomalies of the craniofacial structures.

ETHNIC AND RACIAL FACTORS: Hispanic and Native American children exhibit a significantly greater incidence than Caucasian children, whereas African American children show a significantly lower incidence.

CAREGIVER FACTORS: Children who spend time in day care settings and those who are bottle fed.

hood, with the greatest incidence occurring between birth and seven years of age. The peak period is from birth to two years, a critical time for language acquisition (Howie, Ploussard and Sloyer, 1975; Klein, 1986).

Age is not the only factor related to risk of acquiring middle ear disease. Descriptions of those children most likely to acquire conductive hearing loss associated with otitis media are presented in Table 9.1. Parents and professionals working with children in any of these categories should be alert to signs of middle ear disease and/or changes in hearing so they can actively pursue aggressive medical treatment and avoid potential long-term problems.

Eustachian tube dysfunction is a primary cause of middle ear effusion. When the tube cannot open, air pressure cannot be equalized and negative pressure builds up in the middle ear cavity. In some instances fluid, either clear or infected, accumulates and has no avenue for exit since the Eustachian tube is swollen shut. The presence of fluid interferes with transmission of the sound, causing a hearing loss. Therefore any condition, either permanent or transient, that prevents proper functioning of the tube can result in conductive hearing loss.

Children who are born with head, neck, and craniofacial abnormalities, including those associated with syndromes, are at risk for middle ear disease. Immature and/or improperly functioning palatal muscles may be associated with clefts of the palate. Since the palatal muscles are responsible for pulling open the Eustachian tube, their absence or dysfunction can result in tube dysfunction (Bergstrom, 1986; Jenkins, 1986). Children with this condition as well as those with Down Syndrome have an increased incidence of upper respiratory infection. Children in both groups have poor Eustachian tube function, and their upper respiratory infections are more likely to result in middle ear disease.

Risk for middle ear disease differs across ethnic and racial groups. African American populations demonstrate a significantly lower incidence than Caucasian populations, whereas Hispanic and Native American children have the highest (10-15%) reported occurrence (Todd, 1986). Although some socioeconomic and medical care factors account for disparity of incidence across groups, physiologic group differences are also noteworthy. For example, African Americans and Caucasian Americans have Eustachian tubes that differ according to length, width, and angle of placement (Klein, 1986). Further, some Native American groups have poorer-than-average Eustachian tube function, which is associated with increased episodes of middle ear disease (Beery, et. al., 1980).

Young children who are in day-care centers are exposed to infectious disease at an earlier age than children who remain at home or in multichild home day care. Since such children are at greater risk for otitis media because of their age and have greater exposure to infectious disease, they are more likely to develop otitis media (Klein, 1986). Over the last decade more children have entered day care, either because both their parents are working or they have a single working parent. Because there are more children spending their early years out of the home and with other children, there may be an increase in the number of children with conductive hearing loss. This would increase the number of children in need of special services upon reaching school age.

Infants who are breast fed are less likely to have otitis media than are those who are bottle fed. Infants who breast feed acquire natural immunization from mother's milk, making them less susceptible to infections. The positioning difference between the two types of feeding also has an effect. Bottle-fed babies are typically held in a more prone position, allowing fluid (milk) to pass back toward the Eustachian tube more easily, thus interfering with its normal function. The Eustachian tube is opened by contraction of the palatal muscles, which are exercised more during breast feeding than bottle feeding. A weaker suck is required with bottle feeding resulting in less movement of the palatal muscles. Therefore, Eustachian tube dysfunction (a primary cause of otitis media) is less likely to occur with breast feeding.

Hearing Loss

The type of hearing loss associated with middle ear disease is conductive. Conductive hearing loss is caused by an abnormality in the outer and/or middle ear that typically is treatable medically. Conductive hearing loss can thus be reduced or eliminated when the related disease or structural abnormality is successfully treated.

Otitis media often results in the development of middle ear effusion which can persist even after any infection has been alleviated (Scheidt and Kavanagh, 1986). Children with recurrent middle ear disease can thus have long-term hearing loss, either unilateral or bilateral, that is greater in the low frequencies and varies in degree over time. As the disease progresses from mild to severe, or during its resolution and the course of medication, levels of fluid within the tympanic cavity accumulate and decrease. This change in effusion results in corresponding changes in hearing thresholds—that is, the hearing loss will fluctuate. The changing hearing levels are the causative factors for the auditory and linguistic problems that become obvious themselves in later years.

Auditory Problems

The first indications that there were possible long-term consequences of early onset recurrent middle ear effusion were gleaned from research with laboratory animals. When animals were given a conductive hearing loss during a critical developmental period, differences in the quantity and physiology of neurons within the auditory cortex were noted. Aside from these neurophysiological differences (Webster and Webster, 1977; Webster and Webster, 1979; Webster and Webster, 1980), the animals' psychoacoustic performance when handling a complex auditory signal was poorer than normal (Tess, 1967; Clements and Kelly, 1978).

Such problems have previously been associated with the auditory deprivation caused by long-standing early onset sensorineural hearing loss. However, the report of similar problems occurring when the site of lesion was in the conductive mechanism was a new finding. Based on the tests with animals, clinical concern developed regarding the possibility of conductive hearing loss, especially during periods of language acquisition, causing disruptions in auditory function. Considering the need to cope with acoustically complex signals (speech) on a regular basis, any potential problems would have a profound effect on a child's ability to learn language. The major clinical hypothesis about the effects of early conductive hearing loss is that interference with a clear, consistent speech signal during language acquisition negatively affects the ability to learn the semantic, syntactic and phonological rules of language.

In summary, some children with early onset recurrent fluctuating hearing loss associated with otitis media with effusion demonstrate differences and delays in syntactic development that do not completely resolve over time. Such children may also have persistent speech production and perception difficulties. (Menyuk, 1986).

Communication Problems

The child with conductive hearing loss may demonstrate vowel perception/production errors due to reduced sensitivity to low-frequency elements of speech during the formative years. The residual effects, noted primarily in speech, remain apparent after the hearing deficits have been eliminated, and are most obvious when the episodes have been frequent and have occurred during the period from six months to three years of age. It is less likely that the residual speech effects will be present when the episodes of middle ear disease have occurred only intermittently during this period. Rather than affecting speech, such intermittent fluctuating hearing will result in behavior that is interpreted as inattentive or socially inappropriate.

Adults react to children who have such problems with impatience and annoyance due to the unpredictable and inconsistent behavior they display. Parents may be advised by physicians that associated problems will diminish once the middle ear disease is resolved. This may be true when middle ear disease has been episodic in nature; however, frequently recurring episodes during prime periods of phonological development may produce problems that persist unless addressed through remediation.

Paradoxically, the child with a permanent hearing loss has the advantage of receiving a fairly stable speech signal and can learn how to cope with problems. For example, permanently impaired children realize the difficulty they will have hearing when it is noisy unless they move closer to the speaker. Children with fluctuating hearing acuity may not have had enough experience with the loss to even know that they are not hearing adequately, and thus do not develop the self-help strategies that can enhance communication. Further, the child with a fluctuating hearing loss may be confused due to his/her own inconsistent performance. For example, the child may be a good speller, but due to changing hearing levels gets poor grades on a spelling test because he/she has "misheard" what was said. The child's feelings of self-worth are diminished because he/she understands neither the "problem" nor compensatory strategies.

Auditory Management

Management of children with recurrent middle ear disease and fluctuating hearing loss is quite varied. Medical evaluation and treatment are critical and must be aggressively pursued. Although not their responsibility, it is important for speech, language, and hearing professionals to be familiar with some of the medical options. Antibiotics to directly treat any infection are the most common treatment for middle ear disease. Varying doses of antibiotics can be prescribed on a single-episode basis or as an ongoing prophylaxis, depending on the history of the disease (Shurin, Johnson, and Wegman, 1986).

Since Eustachian tube dysfunction is a primary underlying cause of middle ear effusion, direct treatment procedures may be selected by the physician. Two surgical options, myringotomy and myringotomy with pressure equalizing tubes, ventilate the middle ear cavity, allowing relief of negative pressure. More complete descriptions of the various medical procedures can be found in Bergstrom (1986).

Often physicians base their medical management plan on the degree to which the child's hearing is compromised. For example, if hearing levels remain depressed

Table 9.2 Suggestions for monitoring amplification used in the classroom when children have a history of fluctuating conductive hearing loss.

Attend to changes in auditory behavior

For example,
- child does not respond when his/her name is called,
- child does not hear the answers of other children,
- child does not hear announcements on the P.A. system, or,
- child is "bothered" by doors closing,
- child turns down hearing aid.

Attend to changes in nonauditory behavior

For example,
- child has errors on oral exams,
- child cannot participate in P.E. class,
- child "daydreams" during class, or
- child is "nervous" during class,
- child stays out of social situations.

for prolonged time periods even after antibiotic treatment, the physician may decide that a surgical procedure is necessary. Whereas the immediate goal is to cure the disease, the long-term management plan is to improve the hearing levels.

When medical management does not improve hearing thresholds to within normal limits, or fluctuation in hearing persists, the child must be provided compensatory strategies to access the auditory signal. Some audiologists recommend amplification to improve the child's speech reception in daily listening situations, however, this technique remains controversial for several reasons. When the hearing aid is used only during episodes of depressed hearing levels, a protocol must be established that enables parents and children to know when amplification is necessary. Although careful monitoring of the child's behavior makes implementation of such a controversial protocol possible, it is difficult at best.

If a hearing aid is recommended for full-time use it must be flexible to accommodate the fluctuations in hearing levels. In this case hearing levels must be monitored constantly and a professional must decide on the appropriate changes in hearing aid settings. In both examples, overamplification remains a potential problem that must be considered as seriously as the fluctuation in hearing itself.

Another viable method of amplification is a classroom listening device, either personal or sound field. Since the primary purpose of both types of FM system is to improve the signal-to-noise ratio, either would be a good option for the child who is experiencing problems hearing in noise or other difficult listening conditions. With the personal FM system, as with hearing aids, careful monitoring is required. Table

9.2 illustrates some suggestions for monitoring the use of amplification for children with conductive hearing loss.

When amplification is not the management of choice, other methods of improving the signal-to-noise ratio should be explored. The child must then be near the sound source (requiring some form of preferential seating in the educational setting) and ambient noise levels must be as low as possible. The issues related to difficult listening conditions and classroom modifications are presented in Chapters 2, 5, 6, and 7.

Communication Management

Once identified, those children who have communication deficits as a result of recurrent middle ear disease during formative years require intervention. Efforts to improve speech should go beyond the traditional speech correction procedures and include practice in identifying correct and incorrect productions of others as well as in self-correction.

The problems evidenced by children with a history of fluctuating conductive hearing loss may seem minor compared to those of children who have significant language or phonological disorders. However, they may prevent the child from achieving full academic potential in the junior high and high school years. It is therefore important that these seemingly minor problems be addressed early and aggressively.

Speech-language pathologists may find it difficult to justify the concern and management time for children who are not exhibiting the hearing loss responsible for the problem. Special education administrators are likely to look unfavorably on requests for additional funding and professional time to meet the needs of these "marginally" impaired children. The issue is further complicated by the fact that the available communication assessment tools are ineffective in documenting the deficit areas. The child's problems are seen instead in classroom underachievement.

School subjects that are linguistically based (reading, language arts, social studies, science) are the most difficult during periods of fluctuating hearing and/or with the residual perceptual effects of severe middle ear disease. Real problems occur when children with such deficits must "hear" unfamiliar words, such as names of countries, new vocabulary, and people's names, or perceive the phonetic differences between words, as in reading. Under such conditions they may not "hear" all the elements of the words and sounds, and thus store an incorrect version in their memories. When the words are recalled for expressive or receptive purposes, they do not match the true version and lead to academic errors. For example, during a social studies lesson the teacher said that Pierre is the capital of South Dakota. When that information was incorporated into a test question, a child gave an embarrassingly incorrect answer because he/she heard the teacher say that the capital name was "Beer."

Difficulty in receiving even small segments of the speech signal can have a negative educational impact. If reading is being taught through a phonics approach it is important to detect and discriminate among speech sounds, especially the voiced/voiceless cognates. Therefore when the teacher requests the student to identify the initial sound in the word "pat," he/she silently repeats it as "bat" (exhibiting a voicing error) and responds incorrectly. Management strategies include having the child say the word aloud, thus allowing the teacher an opportunity to hear the student's incorrect rendition and correct it before an answer to the question is given.

Environmental Management

The child with conductive hearing loss is very sensitive to difficult listening conditions. The interference with reception of auditory signals related to changes in the acoustic environment compounds the problems associated with fluctuating and long-term conductive hearing loss. The methods for environmental management presented in Chapters 2, 5, 6, and 7 should thus also be considered for the children with conductive hearing loss.

CHILDREN WITH MILD HEARING LOSS, SPECIFICALLY THOSE CHILDREN WITH PERMANENT HEARING LEVELS BETWEEN 20DB AND 40DB HL.

Incidence

Children with permanent mild sensorineural hearing loss have been identified relatively recently as a group requiring management. An exact incidence rate is not readily available, but when all children with hearing levels (any or all frequencies) greater than 20dB HL are considered, it is estimated to be higher than that at the greater end of the hearing continuum (Matkin, 1988). The average age of identification is thirty-six months for children with mild hearing losses (Matkin, 1988; Malin, Freeman and Hastings, 1976). This late identification results in interference with the child's normal acquisition of language and speech perception categories, which in turn may lead to academic difficulties.

Hearing Loss

By clinical definition mild hearing loss is 40dB or less. It is often limited to the frequency region above 1000 Hz. Since children with mild hearing loss, particularly that of a high frequency configuration, can hear some speech and environmental signals, they are viewed as "hearing" by the naive parent and professional. For ex-

Table 9.3 Behaviors exhibited by infants/toddlers that may indicate the presence of mild hearing loss.

Responds to moderately loud speech and environmental sounds.
Does not respond to soft speech and environmental sounds.
Does not respond when name is called from a distance.
Does not respond when playing with other children.
Does not respond when the television, radio, etc., is on.

ample, hearing part of the speech signal when a parent calls his/her name will allow the child to respond. However, to make good use of the same auditory signal the child must hear it in its entirety. Without repeated access to the complete signal the child cannot learn appropriate categories for speech perception or the morphological markers of spoken English.

Paradoxically, the primary problem for these children is that they hear too well. They respond to auditory signals and develop basic communication skills. Late identification of the hearing loss is exacerbated by the fact that the present neonatal hearing screening guidelines are intended to identify infants with a "significant" (moderate or greater levels between 1000-4000 Hz) hearing loss (Joint Committee on Infant Hearing, 1990). Children with mild hearing losses are therefore not included in the groups typically screened at birth.

Auditory Problems

Although interference with auditory signal reception is less in mild losses than greater ones, there is nonetheless a similar negative effect on acquisition of auditory perceptual skills. Since the child will hear much of what is said or produced in his/her daily listening environment, families do not readily detect the hearing loss.

Table 9.3 demonstrates the type of behaviors that would help parents/caregivers become aware of a mild degree of hearing loss in their children. Often initial reports about such children include comments on their inconsistent responses to sound. Parents know children hear since they startle to loud sounds, turn to footsteps, and "dance" to music. However, these same children do not always respond when their names are called from a distance or attend when there is noise in the background.

To the parents, these responses appear inconsistent, yet careful documentation demonstrates a recognizable pattern. For example, increased distances from the listener (child) to the sound source (speaker) has an adverse effect on the child with mild hearing loss. Although this child can "hear" when close to the speaker, the reduced hearing levels will not accommodate a reduction in sound intensity as the source moves farther away. The child does not hear at a distance but does hear in close proximity, which accounts for the "inconsistent" response.

Negative listening conditions have a greater impact on children with mild hearing loss than on those with normal hearing. Those with mild hearing loss have more difficulty recognizing speech sounds when listening in noise, reverberant conditions or a combination of the two. Their difficulty becomes disproportionately worse as listening conditions become more difficult (Boney and Bess, 1984).

Communication Problems

Children with permanent mild hearing loss are an underserved population. Due to the limited extent of their hearing loss, they are able to detect many of the elements of speech without the assistance of amplification. However, their level of detection is vastly different from that available to children with normal hearing.

Since the speech signal varies in intensity from 35 to 60dB HL, it is obvious that for a child with a 20 to 30dB loss, the softest parts of speech (unvoiced consonants) are barely audible (5 to 10 above threshold), while the louder speech sounds are easily heard (30dB above threshold). Given that spoken language is acquired from listening to audible speech presented in meaningful contexts, it is not surprising that children with very mild degrees of loss demonstrate some delay in phonological and linguistic development. However, since they do hear speech unaided, such children will demonstrate the functional ability to communicate with peers and adults even if the quality and quantity is not commensurate with their same-aged peers. For the student with 30 to 40dB HL losses the softest elements of speech are inaudible, with the louder vowels and voiced consonants being perceived at soft levels. Both of these groups of mildly hearing-impaired children have difficulty accessing the speech of adults during the important language-learning years. The quality of their speech/language reflects the incompleteness of the signal that they have received. Phonological and linguistic deficits may include distortion or absence of the unvoiced sibilants that are used for verb endings, plurality, and possession.

The extreme variability in function evidenced across mildly hearing-impaired students is due to variation in the intensity level of the speech they hear, the listening environment in which they learn language, and the interaction style of the adults providing input. The following are some of the conditions of the living environment that affect the child with mild hearing loss.

Intensity

There is great variability in the habitual loudness level used by parents as they interact with their children. Children whose parents use soft voices will have more difficulty discerning the phonological and linguistic rules in the many examples provided at home. Parents who habitually use loud voices make the voiced elements of speech louder but in no way amplify the unvoiced aspects. Although it becomes easier for their children to alert to speech, the wide discrepancy between the loudest and softest elements of speech makes it particularly difficult to perceive the quiet elements.

Listening Environment

Given equal loudness levels of parental input, the listening environment can further affect the audibility of the signal reaching the child's ears. If the child is learning language in a home that has little interference from background noise (of other children, television, radio), the parent's input regardless of loudness level will more easily reach the child's ears. Competing speech noise is the most deleterious to speech perception; children who are raised with large numbers of siblings frequently have more difficulty discerning who is speaking and what is being said.

Interaction Style

Parental interaction style affects how the parent approaches language stimulation. Parents who, as part of their natural interactions, provide consistent individualized attention to their child firmly establish the association of spoken word and meaning. The process is more difficult when parents rely on "off-the-cuff" interactions to provide meaning for words.

Auditory Management

Management of the mild hearing impairment remains a significant issue even after identification of the hearing loss. For example, debate continues over the necessity and/or appropriateness of amplification for children with such impairment. The argument for fitting the child with amplification as early as possible is the critical need to provide a clear, consistent signal. The major argument against using amplification is the concern of overamplification. That is, the hearing aids will make signals too loud and damage residual hearing.

With so much hearing available, these children should be afforded the opportunity to receive the best possible auditory signal. The audiologist and family should work together to achieve this goal, using the hearing aid evaluation and fitting recommendations suggested in Chapters 2, 5, 6, and 7. Provision of appropriate personal amplification does not ensure easy access to the speech signal in all listening conditions. A wireless FM system may be necessary in difficult listening conditions. The need for an FM system may be even more critical for children with mild hearing loss because they have so much residual hearing. With only hearing aids, in noise and at a distance from the sound source, these children function as if the hearing loss were moderate or even severe.

Although children with mild impairment have more auditory potential than those with greater degrees of hearing loss, they are also much more negatively affected by less-than-optimal listening conditions. Maxon and Brackett (1991) describe a decrease in word recognition when children with mild/moderate hearing loss are confronted with background noise and increased speaker-listener distances, and a corresponding 16% average improvement when an FM unit is used. Actual demonstration of the benefits of the FM system can readily be made by implementing the plan provided in Chapter 7. Use of sound field amplification can be very beneficial for children with mild hearing loss whose hearing levels are better than 30dB HL. It provides a positive signal-to-noise ratio, allowing them to function better in the classroom without fitting a personal device.

Parents of mildly hearing-impaired children are made to feel as though their child's problems are less devastating than those of more severely impaired children. While it is true that the consequences of this degree of loss are less severe, the effect on the family is no less profound. Parents still experience grief for what is lost, denial about the seriousness of the loss, and guilt over having ignored the behaviors that signaled the presence of a hearing loss. Parents of mildly hearing-impaired children find little comfort in support groups that are comprised primarily of parents of children with more severe degrees of hearing loss. The parents may be told they are "lucky" that their child has so much hearing, at a time when these parents feel anything but "lucky."

Communication Management

In addition to increased access to speech through the use of traditional or sound field amplification, the child will need intervention in deficit areas to close the gap between his/her potential and actual speech/language skills. Many speech-language pathologists find it more difficult to work with a child who has what they consider minor deficits than with one who has multiple problems. The issue is to identify the child's marginal vocabulary, syntax, and speech problems and devise intervention strategies that efficiently correct them. Such children, who have the advantage of hearing a consistent signal even with their permanent hearing losses, have an excellent prognosis for making rapid progress when given remediation focused on the deficit areas.

The challenge is to help the parents recognize the seriousness of a seemingly minor hearing loss. When children are able to alert to speech and communicate with adults and other children, it is often difficult to convince parents to accept the overtures of the hearing health care professional. It takes a determined, knowledgeable professional to make the case for having a child wear a visible prosthesis and receive remedial services. As such children mature, they have little difficulty convincing (although erroneously) teachers, parents, and themselves that their hearing aid(s) are providing little benefit in most situations. Since mildly impaired children are able to detect speech, uninformed and inexperienced adults are easily persuaded by this argument. Demonstrating the amount of information missed with unaided functioning may be the only way to convince the family of the benefit of a recommendation.

Children with mild hearing loss may perform within one standard deviation from the norm on most standardized speech and language tests. Yet when their communicative performance is compared to a matched (IQ, SES) group of normally hearing peers, they consistently perform at lower levels. In spite of these documentable differences, few administrators are responsive to parental or professional requests for supportive services that would allow such children to achieve the skills appropriate for their level of intellectual function. As with all degrees of hearing loss, mild loss remains an interfering factor even after intervention has been successful; its effects are everpresent.

Academic Management

When pairs of same-aged normally hearing and mildly hearing-impaired children are matched for intellectual potential and socioeconomic status, the underachievement of the latter group is readily evident. For both reading and math, the children with mild hearing losses do not achieve the same levels of performance as the normally hearing children (Blair, Peterson and Viehweg, 1985). To complicate the issue, this suppression of function occurs even when the hearing-impaired students are functioning at the grade level appropriate for their chronological age. Unless parents are cognizant of this between-group performance discrepancy, they are unable to demand the services their children require to achieve at levels commensurate with their potential.

Academic management of mildly hearing-impaired children includes enhancement of the classroom environment as well as academic support. For children who are so auditorily dependent it is imperative to "hear" what the teacher and other students say. "Hearing" means much more in this context than merely detecting the signal; every effort should be made to access the entire speech signal through classroom amplification, physical modifications, and adaptations in teaching style.

Academic support should vary in frequency according to the student's deficits. Many students need the opportunity to solidify their knowledge by restating the concepts to a tutor and revising the misconceptions that result from "mishearing" the teacher. Others may require a more concentrated preview-review approach in order to absorb new material. "Supporting" the academics requires the student to be in the classroom for the initial presentation of material. Regardless of the frequency of support, care should be taken to remove the child only from nonacademic subjects or unscheduled learning periods, since the time spent in the classroom is critical to his/her success. Juggling the child's need for remediation and for classroom learning requires sensitive, flexible remedial staff.

Environmental Management

Since children with mild hearing loss are so negatively affected by difficult listening conditions, it is important to make physical room modifications when possible. The more that ambient noise levels can be reduced, the better quality will be the auditory signals the child hears. However, such modifications should not be considered the major management component; amplification is the best method of accessing auditory signals and therefore should be the first step.

CHILDREN WITH UNILATERAL HEARING LOSS

Incidence

The number of school-age children with unilateral sensorineural hearing loss greater than a moderate loss in the poor ear is estimated at 2-3/1000. When mild hearing loss in the poorer ear is included, the incidence rises to 13/1000 children (Bess and Tharpe, 1986; Oyler, Oyler and Matkin, 1986). Accurate numbers of preschool and younger children are not known, primarily because of the late age of identification for unilateral loss.

Since the very young unilaterally impaired child responds to normal conversational-level speech as well as soft environmental sounds, there will be little indication in the daily living environment of a hearing problem. As a result, the average age of identification is between five and seven years (Bess and Tharpe, 1986). Children diagnosed at a younger age are usually those whose parents discover the loss by chance. For example, a parent who reads to his daughter at bedtime may realize that she cannot follow the story if he sits on her left side, but has no problem when he sits on the right. It is likely that this father will follow up on the observation by "in-home" testing and then seek professional help.

Another reason for late identification is that language acquisition and speech development follow the expected pattern at the normal rate. Nonauditory signals that may cue bilateral hearing loss are therefore not obvious to the adults in the child's life.

Hearing Loss

Unilateral hearing loss may range from mild to profound in the poor ear, with normal hearing in the other ear. Historically, children with a unilateral impairment have been categorized by the one normal ear and not been considered hearing impaired.

Auditory Problems

A consistent, clear signal in both ears must be present for a child to develop good binaural skills. Those skills include the ability to localize a sound source, readily discriminate speech in noise, and perceive spatial relationships. Children with normal (or equal) hearing in both ears learn to make use of interaural cues in developing binaural skills. They develop skills to perceive the difference in intensity and time of arrival of the signal between the ears. Therefore, if a child does not have fairly equal hearing levels in both ears, he/she will not be readily able to develop such skills.

Children with unilateral hearing loss also demonstrate poor horizontal localization skills, and have difficulty perceiving speech sounds in a background of noise. Maximum interference occurs when speech is directed to the poor ear and the noise is toward the good ear. This situation may be replicated in the classroom if the child is seated with his/her impaired ear toward the teacher and cannot change seats.

Communication Problems

The child with a unilateral hearing loss presents a mixed communicative picture. It is unlikely that he/she was fortunate enough to learn language in a completely quiet environment, without experiencing the deleterious effects of noise and distance on speech reception. As does the child with a fluctuating conductive loss, this child receives an inconsistent speech signal; however, it is due not to the status of hearing, but to the listening environment itself. If the negative environmental conditions that impact on speech reception occur frequently enough, over time the unilaterally impaired child may ultimately exhibit some mild communicative problems. However, more typically the child's academic functioning is compromised due to an inability to hear optimally in the classroom.

The primary nonauditory problem demonstrated by children with unilateral hearing loss is delay in educational progress. Children with unilateral loss are more likely (23-35%) to be retained in grade than their peers with bilaterally normal hearing, who are held back at a rate of 2-3.5%. Further, such children require more special education services—at a rate of at least 40%, when it is less than 10% in the normally hearing population (Bess and Tharp, 1986; Oyler, Oyler, and Matkin, 1986).

When evaluating the speech and language of children with unilateral hearing loss, it is important to determine if the hearing in the good ear has fluctuated in the past. A complete history can be helpful in sifting through factors that may contribute to a language delay. For example, the child who had frequent episodes of middle ear disease and experienced conductive hearing loss in the good ear during language-learning years may exhibit significant language deficits that cannot be attributed to the unilateral hearing impairment present at the time of evaluation.

Auditory Management

There is little controversy about the most appropriate management of children with unilateral hearing loss. Unfortunately, this is because many speech, language, hearing, and educational professionals do not even consider that there may be a need for management. They adhere to the dictum "all you need is one good ear" and do not evaluate the child for special service consideration.

Audiologists are likely to consider amplification as the form of management. Depending on the child's ability to use the impaired ear's residual hearing for speech reception, a CROS or monaural hearing aid may be the amplification of choice. When the hearing loss is severe to profound, the best fit can be achieved with a CROS hearing aid, placing the microphone on the bad ear and the receiver on the good ear. This configuration allows the child to receive the signal from the "bad" side and learn to differentiate between the amplified and unamplified signal to better localize and discriminate speech in noise.

Degree of hearing loss cannot be the sole basis on which to select a hearing aid. Even when poor-ear thresholds are better than severe, there may be cochlear distortion that interferes with discrimination of the speech signal, making it impossible to use monaural amplification in that ear. A CROS hearing aid should be considered in such a case. When the residual hearing is sufficient for reception and perception of speech, a monaural hearing aid or wireless FM system in the poor ear may be the best method of accessing the speech signal.

The choice of amplification cannot be made without a careful evaluation of the child's skills. For monaural amplification the child's binaural performance (good ear unaided and poor ear aided) must not be any worse than when discrimination of the good ear is tested alone. To make this determination the audiologist can assess performance in the sound field with: (1) no amplification; (2) amplification in the poor ear and the good ear plugged; and (3) amplification in the poor ear and the good ear unplugged. There should be no difference in performance between conditions one and three if monaural amplification is to be of any value.

A carefully monitored trial is required to assess the child's ability to use the amplification selected regardless of type. The trial must take place in all the listening environments in which the child functions (home, school, day care, social situations). The FM validation procedure described in Chapter 7 can be modified to assess the benefits of amplification use for the child with unilateral hearing loss.

Some professionals do not consider amplification appropriate management for children with unilateral hearing loss. They suggest environmental modifications instead, to help the child learn to cope with unavoidably difficult listening.

Any auditory management program must include ongoing monitoring of hearing levels and middle ear status of the good ear. Any decrease in good ear hearing levels, whether sensorineural or conductive (associated with middle ear disease), will result in a bilateral hearing loss and completely change the child's skills and problems. Hearing conservation is also crucial to avoid hearing loss resulting from noise exposure. The child with unilateral hearing loss should be encouraged to use ear protection in very noisy listening environments to preserve the good ear's hearing.

Communication Management

Unilaterally impaired children typically demonstrate essentially normal communicative skills unless their better ear has been compromised in the past. However, such children require remedial services to develop compensatory strategies to employ when negative listening conditions exist. Being aware of the need to increase visual access and to request clarification when speech is ambiguous or unintelligible is critical for such students to function in educational settings at levels commensurate with their ability. During management sessions, the professionals can simulate situations in which communicative breakdown typically occurs and demonstrate the use of non-specific requests ("What?" "Say it again") and specific requests ("The name of the dictator is what?".)

Environmental Management

The detrimental effects of noise and reverberation are a primary consideration in managing the child with unilateral hearing loss. If possible, rooms should be physically modified to reduce negative listening conditions and external noise sources should be eliminated or reduced.

If the child is of school age, his/her classroom should be selected for its optimal acoustic environment or be treated. Preferential seating should be recommended, but care must be taken that the child sits with his/her good ear toward the sound source and has flexibility to move as the source moves. Most importantly, when there is a noise source the good ear should be directed away from it.

Children with unilateral hearing loss often have hidden auditory, communication, or academic problems. In-service training regarding problems specific to unilateral impairment and appropriate management strategies must be an IEP component. Administrators, teachers, and other direct service personnel who understand the effect of hearing loss on the child's everyday life in school, home, and social situations will better accept the effort being expended on the child (Bess, Tharpe, and Gibler, 1986).

SUMMARY

The scope of management of hearing-impaired children should be expanded to include children with mild hearing loss, fluctuating conductive hearing loss, and unilateral hearing loss. Each of these conditions interferes with the acquisition of communication skills and impacts on academic performance.

References

Beery, Q.C., Doyle, W.J., Cantekin, E.I., Bluestone, C.D. & Wiet, R.J. (1980). Eustachian tube function in an American Indian population. *Annals of Otology, Rhinology and Laryngology* 89:68, 28-33.

Bergstrom, L. (1986). Otitis media: The surgical approach. In J.F. Kavanagh (Ed.) *Otitis Media and Child Development* (pp.163-175). Parkton, MD: York Press.

Bergstrom, L. (1988). Infectious agents that deafen. In F.H. Bess (Ed.) *Hearing Impairment in Children* (pp. 33-56). Parkton, MD: York Press.

Bess, F.H. & Tharpe, A.M. (1986). Case history data on unilaterally hearing-impaired children. *Ear and Hearing* 7:1,14-19.

Bess, F.H., Tharpe, A.M. & Gibler, A.M. (1986). Auditory performance of children with unilateral sensorineural hearing loss. *Ear and Hearing* 7:1, 20-26.

Blair, J.C., Peterson, M.E. & Viehweg, S.H. (1985). The effects of mild hearing loss on academic performance of young school-age children. *The Volta Review* 87:2, 87-93.

Boney, S. & Bess, F.H. (1984). Noise and reverberation effects on speech recognition in children with minimal hearing loss. Paper presented at the American Speech-Language-Hearing Association, San Francisco, CA.

Clements, M. & Kelly, J.B. (1978). Auditory spatial responses of young guinea pigs (Cavia porcellus) during and after ear blocking. *Journal of Comparative Physiological Psychology* 92, 34-44.

Howie, V.M., Ploussard, J.H. & Sloyer, J. (1975). The "otitis-prone" condition. *American Journal of Diseases of Children* 129, 676-678.

Jenkins, J.J. (1986). Cognitive development in children with recurrent otitis media: Where do we stand? In J.F. Kavanagh (Ed.) *Otitis Media and Child Development* (pp.211-222). Parkton, MD: York Press.

Joint Committee on Infant Hearing: *Draft Position Statement on the High Risk Register for Hearing Loss,* 1990.

Klein, J.O. (1986). Risk factors for otitis media in children. In J.F. Kavanagh (Ed.) *Otitis Media and Child Development* (pp. 45-51). Parkton, MD: York Press.

Malkin, S.F., Freeman, R.D. & Hastings, J.O. (1976). Psychosocial problems of deaf children and their families: A comparative study. *Audiology, Hearing and Education* 2, 21-29.

Matkin, N.D. (1988). Re-evaluating our approach to evaluation: Demographics are changing—are we? In F.H. Bess (Ed.) *Hearing Impairment in Children* (pp. 101-111). Parkton, MD: York Press.

Maxon, A.B. & Brackett, D. (1991). FM use for children with mild hearing loss: Necessity or luxury. *Proceedings of 6th International SHHH Convention.* 53-56.

Menyuk, P. (1986). Predicting speech and language problems with persistent otitis media. In J.F. Kavanagh (Ed.) *Otitis Media and Child Development* (pp.83-98). Parkton, MD: York Press.

Oyler, R.F., Oyler, A.L. & Matkin, N.D. (1986). Unilateral hearing loss: Demographics and educational impact. Paper presented at American Speech-Language-Hearing Association Convention, Detroit, MI.

Scheidt, P.C. & Kavanagh, J.F. (1986). Common terminology for conditions of the middle ear. In J.F. Kavanagh (Ed.) *Otitis Media and Child Development* (pp. 15-17). Parkton, MD: York Press.

Shurin, P.A., Johnson, C.E. & Wegman, D.L. (1986). Medical aspects of diagnosis and prevention of otitis media. In J.F. Kavanagh (Ed.) *Otitis Media and Child Development* (pp. 60-69). Parkton, MD: York Press.

Tess, R.C. (1967). The effects of early auditory restriction in the rat on adult duration discrimination. *Journal of Auditory Research 7*, 195-207.

Todd, N.W. (1986). High risk populations for otitis media. In J.F. Kavanagh (Ed.) *Otitis Media and Child Development* (pp. 52-59). Parkton, MD: York Press.

Webster, D.B. & Webster, M. (1977). Neonatal sound deprivation affects brainstem auditory nuclei. *Archives of Otolaryngology 103*, 392-406.

Webster, D.B. & Webster, M. (1979). Effects of neonatal conductive hearing loss on brainstem auditory nuclei. *Annals of Otology, Rhinology, and Laryngology 88*, 684-688.

Webster, D.B. & Webster, M. (1980). Mouse brainstem auditory nuclei development. *Annals of Otology, Rhinology, and Laryngology 89*, 254-256.

10

Team Approach

INTRODUCTION

Managing hearing-impaired children requires the interaction of families, children, and a variety of professionals. The specific devices, procedures, and methods for developing an appropriate plan (either IFSP or IEP) have been discussed in previous chapters. However, issues remain related to coordination, communication among team members, advocating for student's rights, and in-service training—the foundation on which the plan is built.

The previous chapters repeatedly stressed the widely varying communicative, social, and academic effects of congenital and early onset hearing loss, which cannot be predicted by knowing the degree and configuration of the loss. The deficit areas span the domains of several health care and education professions. To ensure that all areas of need are appropriately assessed and managed, a multidisciplinary team approach should be used. Such a model is mandated by P.L. 99-457 and can easily be incorporated into the regulations of P.L. 94-142. Team management is thus an effective format regardless of age or setting.

The members of the team should include professionals with expertise in the deficit areas exhibited by the student. Since the child's profile changes over time, so should the composition of the team. Table 10.1 lists the professionals who can contribute to the management of hearing impaired students. However, rather than their degrees or credentials, the professionals' specific competencies, skills, and knowledge should be the basis for team inclusion. Professionals whose strengths accommodate the needs of the particular child will thus be the ones providing services.

The role of the aural rehabilitation (AR) specialist changes over time as the child's world broadens to include sources of input other than the immediate family (Table 10.2). The AR specialist concentrates initially on establishing functional communication skills by enhancing the interaction between caregiver and child. As the child approaches age three, the professional and parent must explore the available educational options and decide which one best meets his/her specific needs. Although the mainstream nursery school provides organized social/educational opportunities, the child will be unable to access the rich verbal input unless modifications are implemented. The specialist must prepare not only the child for the

Table 10.1   The role of individuals who should be considered for inclusion on the multidisciplinary planning team for a child with hearing loss.

Individual	Role
Audiologist	Provide information about: hearing loss, personal amplification, classroom amplification, auditory needs, auditory management, listening conditions.
Speech-Language Pathologist	Provide information about: communication abilities, communication management, effects of hearing loss on speech and language, effects of skills on academics, educational management.
Teacher of the Hearing Impaired	Provide information about: academic needs, adapting curriculum, teaching children with hearing loss educational management.
Regular Education Teacher	Provide information about: regular education curriculum, accommodating special needs, classroom demands.
Special Education Teacher	Provide information about: academic support services, accommodating special needs.
Parent(s)	Provide information about: the child's hearing, the child's communication, family expectations, the child's potential.
Psychologist	Provide information about: child's intellectual potential, social adjustment.
Tutor	Provide information about: academic support.

Table 10.2 The changing role of aural rehabilitation specialist over time, with the number of X's representing the intensity of the contact.

	Child	*Family/Parent Caregiver*	*Education*
Infant/ Toddler	XXXXX	XXXXX	
Preschool Mainstream	XXX	XXX	XXX
Preschool Self-Contained	XX	X	XXXX
School Age Mainstream	XXX	X	XXX
School Age Self-Contained	X	X	XXXX

experience, but also the educational setting for the child. The role of the AR remains critical throughout the school career of the student in a mainstream track. If the child enters a self-contained class, the primary responsibility for language and speech acquisition is transferred to the special educator, with individualized support services provided by the AR specialist. The same pattern continues throughout the school years, with the AR specialist playing a major role with the mainstreamed student, and a less intense role with the child educated in a specialized self-contained class.

The team approach is most effective if one person is responsible for organizing the plan and ensuring that it is implemented. A case manager should be designated, whose role includes: (1) coordination and integration of all services; (2) knowledge of service delivery options and consultants; (3) provision of in-service training to other professionals, parents, peers, and community professionals; (4) advocacy; and (5) provision of direct services. The designated professional should be the team member most knowledgeable about hearing impairment and its effects in the particular child.

As the child's management and educational placement change, so will the primary case manager. In mainstream settings, the professional providing direct remediation, either the speech-language pathologist, teacher of the hearing impaired, or audiologist, tends to be the best informed about the child's functional capability in a variety of social and academic situations. Once a self-contained placement is chosen, the classroom teacher may be the logical choice for case manager.

PROFESSIONAL ADVOCACY

The professionals on the team should view themselves as partners with the parents in developing an appropriate program. In that capacity they: (1) inform parents about the child's strengths and weaknesses; (2) recommend appropriate and effective services to address the deficit areas; and (3) help parents understand strategies for effective advocacy.

The case manager is responsible for presenting the hearing-impaired child in a realistic yet positive light to other school personnel. This includes providing in-service to all teachers and ancillary personnel who are involved in the child's education. For example, helping the school staff accept the use of an FM unit requires tactful yet persuasive arguments from the resident expert.

Unfortunately, a more typical scenario places the parents and professionals on opposing sides. For example, the parents may have learned on their own about services potentially appropriate for their child, but are confronted with school personnel who do not even consider their opinions. Often parents have to bring in outside experts to testify about the efficacy of their recommendations before the team will recognize their worth. Much of the controversy can be avoided if school personnel are willing to investigate a variety of options and services for the child.

PARENT ADVOCACY

If parent education programs have been successful, they have given parents the knowledge necessary to advocate for their child in educational and social situations. However, unless they have practiced strategies to effectively present such information, parents may experience difficulty in getting professionals to comply with their requests. Some parents naturally adopt an attitude that is informative and nonconfrontational. They understand when to stand their ground and when to compromise. They have researched the issues under consideration and provide written and oral testimony to support their arguments. Such an informed approach becomes especially important when one program is being compared to another.

Parents who have made themselves indispensable to the school are more likely to achieve positive results at their child's planning meeting. Such parents understand the need to make their presence felt at Board of Education meetings, as parent advocates on special education committees, at school activities, and at PTA meetings.

Parents may find themselves in meetings where they have to defend a programming decision for their child. The issues involved can be divided into class placement, service delivery, and communicative modality.

Services

Often schools and families enter potentially confrontational discussions over the frequency and quality of the support services available through the school system.

Although the law provides for free and appropriate education, it does not require that the "most appropriate" option be selected. It becomes the parents' responsibility to convince the school that the funds and effort expended are an investment in the child's future—the provision of appropriate support services now ensures that less money will be needed for special education services in the future. This argument is especially salient during the preschool years.

Once the services are selected, the issue of who will provide them (qualifications and experience) must be resolved. If the child's needs are sufficiently specialized to require a specially trained professional, that should not be an area of compromise. Another area for discussion is how the services will be provided. If the student is mainstreamed, an effort should be made to allow the student to remain in the classroom for all the academic subject areas, instead of pulling him/her out for remedial work. Parents should argue that if the student is held responsible for the information presented during the classroom lessons he/she should have the advantage of hearing it.

Class Placement

Class placement, such as moving the child to a less restrictive environment, may be initiated by the school, especially if it is interested in bringing children back to their own school districts from out-of-town placements. However, parents are often reluctant to give up the nurturing self-contained classroom for the competitive, highly verbal mainstream class.

Communicative Modality

The most fundamental discussion between parents and educators concerns the parents' choice of communicative modality for their child. If they have made their initial decision based on an informed choice, and if that decision has been reevaluated and validated over time by both parents and professionals, this discussion should be perfunctory. If the parents had not sufficiently considered the issue at the time of identification, they will have to get a professional opinion to support their proposals.

Often parents have to readdress the modality issue several times during the child's educational life—at the start of preschool, the beginning of kindergarten, the transition from elementary school to junior high/middle school, the transition to high school, and at exit to postsecondary programs. The evaluations and follow-up planning meetings that typically occur at these transition points act as a catalyst for addressing difficult and controversial issues. School professionals usually want assurance that another educational placement or communicative modality would not be more beneficial. For the mainstreamed child, their concern is that he/she is not getting as much out of the classroom presentation as the normally hearing children. Although this may be true, it must be weighed against the lower demand and content level of the self-contained environment.

PARENT ADVOCACY STRATEGIES

Avoid criticizing another program or the professionals in it. Parents will receive greater acceptance if they discuss areas in which programs differ and stress the necessity of particular items for their child. For example, if an alternative program offers structured speech work as a classroom activity, the parents should emphasize their child's need for individual sessions to learn skills that differ from those introduced in the class.

Identify those issues for which there is no compromise. If there are certain basic requirements without which the child cannot function in a particular setting, parents must insist that they appear on the IEP. They can avoid a stalemate if they are prepared to compromise on other issues that can be modified without jeopardizing the integrity of the program. For nonnegotiable issues the parents must be willing to go to due process if a consensus cannot be reached at the IEP meeting. For example, if a hearing-impaired child is fortunate enough to have achieved age- and grade-appropriate skills, the parent will have to insist on continued academic support in order for the child to retain this level over time.

Present the child in a positive light. Parents should stress what the child can offer the class, rather than what the program needs to do for the child. Comments such as "he has a wonderful sense of humor" or "she has a dramatic flair" describe what the child can do. Conversely, saying that the child has delayed language skills and must be required to talk, e.g., to say something when the juice is passed, only points out his/her differences. This is especially important for the child being considered for a mainstream educational setting. If he/she has extensive "special" needs, then a classroom teacher who has never worked with hearing-impaired children will be quick to suggest an alternative placement where "special" attention is possible, e.g., in a class with reduced numbers of children.

Indicate that the classroom teacher is not solely responsible for the child. The classroom teacher may be concerned about his/her limited knowledge of hearing loss. As a member of the team, the teacher will receive in-service training and ongoing support from experienced personnel. Having such support structures can help a teacher accept the hearing-impaired child.

PARENT ADVOCACY PRACTICE

Members of an active parent group can critique each other as they role-play these confrontational situations. It can be informative to hear how other people might introduce their child to a nursery school teacher, request services as their child enters school, or request a change in placement. Modelling these situations allows parents to make their mistakes in front of a sympathetic audience and to benefit from the mistakes of others.

IN-SERVICE TRAINING

In-service training fills an informational and experiential void in the education of regular school personnel (Maxon, 1991). The resident expert (case manager) is typically assigned the responsibility of informing the regular school staff about the particular needs of the hearing-impaired student. In some instances, more specific training may be available for a fee from professionals at a hearing health care facility, university clinic, or regional program for the hearing impaired.

The audience for workshops will vary, depending on the breadth of the program and the needs of the school personnel. The teachers who have direct contact with the student are the primary recipients of information. Not only do they need to understand the general effects of hearing loss, but also how the hearing loss has specifically impacted on the particular student. This requires a review of the student's multidisciplinary evaluations and interpretation of the results relative to school performance and social interaction. Management suggestions evolve out of such an analysis. Inexperienced teachers will also need assistance in making their classroom lectures fully accessible to the student.

The second level of in-service training addresses school staff who have intermittent contact with the hearing-impaired student, such as the clerical staff, school nurse, janitors, and lunchroom attendants. While their involvement does not impact dramatically on academic performance, their understanding assists in the child's full acceptance in all aspects of school life.

A third group, often ignored, comprises the classmates of the hearing-impaired student. When the student is new to the school or class, having an open classroom discussion of hearing impairment and amplification equipment can reduce negative comments and increase social integration. Some hearing-impaired children will appreciate the opportunity to talk about their condition in front of their peers, and may describe it as unique rather than negative. Others prefer to keep their differences to themselves, and choose to be absent from such a discussion. For elementary school children, it is beneficial to pair the discussion with a unit on senses. In the older grades, biology class provides a forum for explaining in detail the structure of the ear, how it functions, and the consequences of hearing impairment. A follow-up exercise may include experiencing the effects of hearing impairment with earplugs and writing about its effects on interaction and daily routines. Increasing the awareness of classmates is the surest way to diffuse the mystery of hearing impairment.

Informal training occurs on a regular basis with the student's primary teachers. The designated trainer observes in the classroom, following up with suggestions on how to facilitate interaction between the hearing-impaired student and his/her classmates and teachers. Information exchanges should be directly related to questions asked by the teachers. If such questions concern the student's inconsistent attention and responsiveness, the teacher needs information about the effect of classroom noise and speaker-listener distance on perception of speech. Specific suggestions should focus on maintaining close proximity between the teacher and student, especially when there is interfering noise.

The timing of the in-service training varies according to the function of the workshop. Orientation for primary teachers should occur before the first day of school; the teacher will thus be able to build in the modifications that are necessary to ensure that the hearing-impaired student will have access to teacher input while he/she is preparing the classroom for the beginning of school. Routine follow-up visits should be scheduled at the teacher's convenience. Although formal workshops are scheduled at various times during the school year, the earlier in the year one occurs, the more positive its impact on the student.

COORDINATION

There is a critical need for communication between clinical service providers and teachers in the school or early intervention program. Merely reiterating that there is a need to keep all the involved professionals informed is not useful unless specific strategies for accomplishing this task are implemented.

During the preschool years, the parents of children in mainstream nursery schools act as liaison between the remedial service providers and the classroom teacher. Unless the rehabilitation is provided on site at the nursery school, there is little opportunity for the special and regular education personnel to interact. Telephone contact is a useful alternative to maintaining updated contact between the two sites. In reality, it is the information transmitted by the parents that becomes the basis of day-to-day program modifications. Strategies such as obtaining the lesson plans prior to the week in which they are taught or obtaining the overall curriculum before school starts can be effective in targeting similar topics or concepts in both the rehabilitation and education environments.

In preschool classes for the hearing-impaired, coordination becomes the responsibility of the interested parent and the classroom teacher. If remedial services are conducted outside of the regular classroom, a vehicle for transmitting information between professional and parent should be established. A notebook transported between home and school can be an effective method of informing the parent about daily goals, objectives, progress, and suggested home activities.

For the school-age child, the responsibility for making the initial contact with the classroom teacher lies with the case manager, who has the most information about his/her strengths, weaknesses, and needs. Most teachers have very little time to spend on this kind of coordination; it therefore behooves the case manager to identify a strategy that provides efficient transmission of routine information. The burden for maintaining the designated procedures also falls to the case manager. Even the most cooperative teachers will discontinue the coordination effort if they feel that their information is not important enough to warrant a response. Thus, each entry from the teacher requires a comment from the case manager.

In optimal situations, coordination time is written into the IEP. One period a week should be designated for planning, in order to identify deficit areas, review schedules of tests and assignments, and preview the next week's subject areas. When the child has multiple teachers for the main academic subjects, coordination obviously becomes much more difficult.

Observation is likely to be one-sided; it is usually easier for the support service providers than for the classroom teacher to observe the child during classroom activities. (Few classroom teachers have a substitute teacher or aide readily available to fill in for them.) Even intermittent viewing of the child as he/she applies skills during classroom lectures or social interaction can be revealing to the support service providers. The reports of such visits can be the basis for discussion at regularly scheduled interdisciplinary planning meetings and/or entered in the notebook.

SUMMARY

Due to the wide variation in educational, communicative and social needs of children with hearing loss no one program or service delivery model can be applied to all situations. A carefully designed and monitored individualized education program requires input from a team comprised of school professionals and parents. Close coordination among team members ensures the success of these highly individualized programs.

Reference

Maxon, A.B. (1991). Implementing an in-service training program. In M. Ross (Ed.) *Hearing-Impaired Children in the Mainstream.* Parkton, MD: York Press.

Appendix

Daily amplification troubleshooting protocols were described by Ross, Brackett, and Maxon (1991). The following is an adaptation of their descriptions.

Equipment Needed

a. Battery tester. It should be calibrated in volts, and accommodate 9-volt batteries.

b. Listening stethoscope. It couples the amplification to the listener's ears. When evaluating the earmold or tone hook of ear-level instruments, the stethoscope tubing is used. To accommodate snap-on (button) transducers, the tubing is removed and the transducer snapped directly to stethoscope earpieces.

c. Personal earmold. An examiner's personal earmold or "stock earmold" can be used for troubleshooting. Thereafter, a snap-on earmold is used for button transducers and an adapter for ear-level fittings.

d. Earmold cleaner. Earmold antiseptic, or warm water and mild soap, are used to clean earmolds. Pipe cleaners, toothpicks, and an air syringe are used to remove wax from a clogged earmold.

e. Supplies. Batteries, cords, and transducers should be stocked to replace inoperable parts.

Personal Hearing Aids

1. Visual inspection.

a. Case. Examine the case for dents or other disfigurements. Physical damage does not always indicate electroacoustic problems, but may be associated with a malfunctioning instrument. Examine the battery compartment for corrosion and improper battery contact. The battery terminals may be bent, corroded, or missing, causing inadequate electrical connection.

b. Controls. Deactivate the hearing aid telephone coil ("T" switch) so the microphone can function. Verify correct positioning of all external controls (e.g., tone and output).

c. Tone hook. Examine the tone hook of ear-level hearing aids for cracks and security of connection. With a screw-on connection the threads may be stripped and the tone hook may need to be replaced.

d. Connecting cords. Examine the cords (body, CROS, bone conduction hearing aids) to determine whether the insulation has been stripped, causing a short circuit or broken connection. Check the cord prongs on both ends to determine if they fit snugly into the outlets and can be fully inserted.

e. Transducers. Examine transducers (body or bone conduction hearing aids) for cracks or dents.

f. Earmolds. Examine all types of earmolds, being aware of any special modifications such as venting. Inspect the sound bore for wax that may be clogging it. Clean earmolds with a mild soap and warm water. Examine earmold tubing for cracks, crimping, and inflexibility. Inspect earmolds for lacerations and discolorations.

2. Battery check.

Prior to the listening inspection, test batteries for proper voltage readings. Replace if "low".

3. Earmold insertion.

Observe when the child inserts the earmold, being sure it is fully seated in the concha, with no feedback or discomfort.

4. Listening inspection.

Use the hearing aid stethoscope or personal earmold. Listen for distortion, noise, intermittent signals, or inadequate amplification. When possible, listen at the volume level used by the child (not recommended for high-gain hearing aids).

a. Volume. Rotate volume control from the off position to a higher level. The signal should increase gradually with slight rotation. Listen for static or other interference when the volume control is turned.

b. Cords. Manipulate the cords and listen to changes in sound amplification. Replace cords if there is an intermittent signal or static.

c. Sound quality. Listen for a clear and undistorted signal. Consider tone settings that make the sound "tinny" or "low pitched."

d. Earmold. Listen via the child's earmold to ensure it is not clogged.

Traditional (Self-contained) FM Systems

1. Visual Inspection. Follow the guidelines presented above when troubleshooting a traditional FM system. Check both the receiver and the transmitter.

a. Receiver (child's unit). Inspect right and left channels for cords, transducers, earmolds, and settings.

b. Transmitter (teacher's microphone). Check antenna for cracks and breaks that interfere with the transmission of the FM signal. Inspect cord and connections of remote microphone when part of the transmitter.

c. Batteries. Check battery compartments on receiver and transmitter for loose contacts and broken wires.

2. Listening inspection.

a. Receiver. Manipulate cords and transducers. Listen for interference with the conduction and/or quality of the sound. Turn off FM transmitter and check linearity of the volume control, amplification level, and quality of the environmental microphone signal. Check each channel (right, left) individually.

b. Transmitter. The FM transmitter must be checked in conjunction with the FM receiver, requiring a second examiner. Listen with FM-only reception (turn off the environmental microphones) and with both the FM and environmental microphones activated. Ensure signal arriving at the FM microphone is louder than those arriving at the environmental microphones. Have second examiner speak into the transmitter at ten feet away while first examiner speaks into the environmental microphones. Check each channel (right, left) separately.

Personal FM Systems

First troubleshoot hearing aids that couple to FM receiver.

1. Visual inspection. Use inspections described above. Pay specific attention to:

a. Direct audio-input cords.

b. Direct audio-input shoe/boot.

c. Induction (neck) loop for telecoil reception.

d. Telephone switch on the hearing aid.

2. Listening inspection. Use the listening conditions described for the traditional FM systems. Be careful when:

a. Listening via a loop coupling. Wear the loop and hold hearing aid at ear level to determine whether signal is strong enough. Move the hearing aid and listen for changes in the strength and quality of the signal.

b. There is direct audio input coupling. Check each boot/shoe and cords individually. Listen for interference related to the connection.

c. Using either coupling. Deactivate hearing aid microphones when listening to FM-only transmission.

d. Batteries. Most units have rechargeable batteries. Monitor length of time the batteries hold a charge. Nine-volt batteries can be replaced by the nickel cadmium type.

Index